Providing diabetes care in general practice

Acknowledgements

My grateful thanks go to the following people for their help and support in the production of *Providing Diabetes Care in General Practice*:

Judith North for checking every word

Charles Fox for 'comments from a diabetologist'

Norman How for 'comments from general practice'

Michael Hall for writing the Foreword

Richard Warner for encouraging me to write the book

My family for putting up with it

Very special thanks go to Katherine Kennedy for her dedication in providing a fine manuscript and without whom the book could not have been produced at all.

Finally, I would like to thank people with diabetes and my colleagues in general practice and diabetes care in Sheffield for their support over many years and who have, through their shared experience, made an invaluable contribution to this book.

Contents

Part 1 Diabetes: an overview
1 Responsibilities of those involved in the provision of diabetes care 3
2 Educational needs of the team 9
3 Diabetes mellitus in the United Kingdom 16

Part 2 Providing diabetes care
4 The diabetes service in general practice 33
5 The symptoms of diabetes mellitus 45
6 Providing the service 61
7 The treatment of non-insulin dependent diabetes mellitus 72
8 Drug and insulin therapy 82
9 Aspects of culture relating to diabetes care 99
10 Control of blood glucose levels 106
11 Eye care and screening 119
12 Foot care and surveillance 130
13 Education for self-management 144
14 Living with diabetes: information requirements 153
15 Monitoring and audit of practice diabetes care 165
16 Resources for the provision of diabetes care 171

Part 3 About diabetes
17 Diabetes mellitus: a history of the condition 179
18 Insulin dependent diabetes (IDDM) 182
19 Non-insulin dependent diabetes mellitus (NIDDM) 185
20 Other categories of diabetes 189
21 Other causes of diabetes – secondary diabetes 192
22 The complications of diabetes 196
23 Conclusion 206

Appendices
I British Diabetic Association – unit membership for general practice 209
II The rights and roles of people with diabetes – 'what care to expect' 210
III St Vincent Declaration recommendations for the care of children 214
IV Department of Health requirements 217
V British Diabetic Association recommendations for the management of diabetes in primary care 219
Index 223

Foreword

Every now and again the practice of medicine takes a great step forward. Those of us involved at the moment are part of that advance and take pleasure in it.

It may be the development of a vaccine or the discoveryof a new drug.

The new organisation of the health service in Britain has confused and at the same time has increased the work-load and often exhausted and stressed the professionals involved. In spite of all this I believe the new systems of care for our patients present great opportunities which can improve quality of life and reduce the complications of many of the common chronic conditions which afflict man at the end of the 20th century.

The system of diabetes care is about to become one of those important central advances. The discovery of insulin was rightly heralded as one of the century's great medical events. It brought life to many who had not expected it but because people now survive, it inevitably meant that health professionals now have to manage large numbers of people, some with long-term complications which could not have been envisaged.

We know that successful management depends upon the good glycaemic control and the detection of the earliest signs of complications. The problem has always been of trying to monitor all those with diabetes. The difficulty of keeping track of so many people through a hospital based service, especially when so many people with diabetes rarely attend hospital is well known.

Now at last we are to link responsibility for regular monitoring of people with diabetes into the population registers of general practitioners. The new arrangements for diabetes care in general practice have taken account of the best professional advice in both specialist and primary care. It will allow GPs, practice nurses and other professionals in the primary health care teams the opportunity to become central players in diabetes care.

I welcome this delightfully written book. It is the complete guide for the primary health care team. It will help all those wishing to plan or participate in a diabetes care programme and its well referenced index makes it quick and easy to use.

Dr Michael Hall, General Practitioner
Joint Vice Chairman of the British Diabetic Association

Introduction

Increasingly, the primary care team in general practice has become more aware and involved in the care of people with diabetes mellitus. From 1 July 1993, diabetes will enter into the category of disease management with service provision to be agreed between Health District purchasers and providers.

The purpose of this book is to provide a practical and helpful guide to the care of people with diabetes by the team in general practice. The book is set out for easy use in the working situation and is divided into three main parts.

Part 1 *Diabetes – an overview* sets the scene, including the roles and educational needs of the primary care team and the organisation of diabetes services in the United Kingdom.

Part 2 *Providing diabetes care* describes how to set up and run the service in general practice.

Part 3 *About diabetes* provides further information about the condition and associated complications.

Further information relating to guidelines and recommendations are included in the Appendices. Throughout the book, summaries are used for quick reference.

The St Vincent Declaration was agreed in October 1989. The Declaration, endorsed by all European countries, set out goals for the future planning of diabetes care and the implementation of effective measures for the reduction of the complications of the condition. Although particular to diabetes, the St Vincent Declaration coincided with the proposals for change identified in the 1990 Department of Health *Health of the Nation* document.

The process by which the goals of St Vincent will be achieved is by greater involvement of people with diabetes in their own care and with all health care professionals working together to reduce the burden of this complex condition, the nature of which is described by a person living with diabetes.

Living with diabetes – Brian's story

"I have been diabetic for 30 years. To begin with I was told I was a mild case, put on tablets and a strict diet and told 'not to worry, we can keep you alive for years yet'. Not particularly encouraged by this attitude, I decided I could take care of myself. I read several books about diabetes, because in those days not such a lot was known about the condition and there was not the help available by having someone to talk to or advise.

Over the years my condition deteriorated, mostly I suppose because I tried to ignore it. I took my tablets, but diet-wise I was not very 'wise'. Gradually my eyesight deteriorated and it is now necessary for me to attend the Eye Clinic regularly and to have periodic laser treatment on both eyes. Because laser treatment is now used I am fortunate that I can still see but some diabetics do go blind. My feet and legs have also become a problem and now my mobility is very much impaired. I have learned over the years to live with my illness and now I am much more careful about my diet, but I still have my likes and dislikes.

During the last year I have had three spells in hospital, two because my feet have not been alright and one because of my eyes. I have found that health care professionals as a whole can be very ignorant about the diabetic's needs, simply thinking that they must have a strict routine and can only eat certain things. Definitely no sugar and so many blood tests each day that by the end of a week your fingers are so sore you do not know what to do with them and then multiply that lot for a year – I doubt you would have any finger ends left. They do not seem to think the diabetic knows anything about his own condition. I know what I can eat within reason and now that I am on insulin, I know how to adjust it should my blood sugar rise.

Diabetes is not an easy condition to live with, not just from my point of view but from a family point of view. I find I tire much more easily and because of the problems with my legs and feet, I cannot walk far. Consequently a lot of the things we did as a family we cannot now do. It restricts us an awful lot as far as activities are concerned and from my wife's angle can be very frustrating for her as well. When I have had problems both with my eyes and feet, I have had to sit in one room for several weeks and life becomes very tedious. It is then you need a lot of support both from your family and medical people who understand the problems and can come up with practical help both for the diabetic himself and his family."

Brian's story gives an insight into living with diabetes mellitus. In it he clearly identifies his own difficulties which have progressed over many years and affect not only his life but that of his wife and family. In listening to him, the goals and targets recommended in the St Vincent Declaration take on a very special meaning.

The St Vincent Declaration

Diabetes Care and Research in Europe
The Saint Vincent Declaration

Representatives of Government Health Departments and patients' organisations from all European countries met with diabetes experts under the aegis of the Regional Offices of the World Health Organisation and the International Diabetes Federation in St Vincent, Italy on October 10-12, 1989. They unanimously agreed upon the following recommendations and urged that they should be presented in all countries throughout Europe for implementation.

"Diabetes mellitus is a major and growing European health problem, a problem at all ages and in all countries. It causes prolonged ill-health and early death. It threatens at least ten million European citizens.

It is within the power of national Governments and Health Departments to create conditions in which a major reduction in this heavy burden of disease and death can be achieved. Countries should give formal recognition to the diabetes problem and deploy resources for its solution. Plans for the prevention, identification and treatment of diabetes and particularly its complications – blindness, renal failure, gangrene and amputation, aggravated coronary heart disease and stroke – should be formulated at local, national and European regional levels. Investment now will earn great dividends in reduction of human misery and in massive savings of human and material resources.

General goals and five-year targets listed below can be achieved by the organised activities of the medical services in active partnership with diabetic citizens, their families, friends and workmates and their organisations; in the management of their own diabetes and the education for it; in the planning, provision and quality audit of health care; in national, regional and international organisations for disseminating information about health maintenance; in promoting and applying research.

General goals for people – children and adults – with diabetes
- Sustained improvement in health experience and a life approaching normal expectation in quality and quantity.
- Prevention and cure of diabetes and of its complications by intensifying research effort.

Five-year targets
Elaborate, initiate and evaluate comprehensive programmes for detection and control of diabetes and of its complications with self-care and community support as major components.

Raise awareness in the population and among health care professionals of the present opportunities and the future needs for prevention of the complications of diabetes and of diabetes itself.

Organise training and teaching in diabetes management and care for people of all ages with diabetes, for their families, friends and working associates and for the health care team .

Ensure that care for children with diabetes is provided by individuals and teams specialised both in the management of diabetes and of children, and that families with a diabetic child get the necessary social, economic and emotional support.

Reinforce existing centres of excellence in diabetes care, education and research. Create new centres where the need and potential exist.

Promote independence, equity and self-sufficiency for all people with diabetes – children, adolescents, those in the working years of life and the elderly.

Remove hindrances to the fullest possible integration of the diabetic citizen into society.

Implement effective measures for the prevention of costly complications
• Reduce new blindness due to diabetes by one third or more.
• Reduce numbers of people entering end-stage diabetic renal failure by at least one third.
• Reduce by one half the rate of limb amputations for diabetic gangrene.
• Cut morbidity and mortality from coronary heart disease in the diabetic by vigorous programmes of risk factor reduction.
• Achieve pregnancy outcome in the diabetic woman that approximates that of the non-diabetic woman.

Establish monitoring and control systems using state of the art information technology for quality assurance of diabetes health care provision and for laboratory and technical procedures in diabetes diagnosis, treatment and self-management.

Promote European and international collaboration in programmes of diabetes research and development through national, regional and WHO agencies and in active partnership with diabetes patients organisations.

Take urgent action in the spirit of the WHO programme, 'Health for All' to establish joint machinery between WHO and IDF, European Region, to initiate, accelerate and facilitate the implementation of these recommendations.''

At the conclusion of the St. Vincent meeting, all those attending formally pledged themselves to strong and decisive action in seeking implementation of the recommendations on their return home.

The St Vincent Declaration Joint Department of Health/British Diabetic Association Task Force

In July 1992, the Department of Health announced that a Joint Task Force with the British Diabetic Association would be set up, with terms of reference to include advising on which aspects of the St Vincent Declaration need to be addressed, assessing their relative priority and providing detailed advice on a programme of action required to implement agreed priority areas.

Part 1 Diabetes: an overview

1 Responsibilities of those involved in the provision of diabetes care

The general practitioner

The general practitioner takes overall clinical responsibility for the provision of care. In addition, the GP, as an employer, is bound by the code of conduct of the General Medical Council. In employing practice nurses, the doctors 'must be satisfied that the person to whom they delegate duties is competent to carry out (such) treatments and procedures'.

The practice nurse

The practice nurse (or community nurse, if involved), is professionally accountable for any nursing service provided, as laid down by the UKCC. In a specialist subject, such as diabetes, where particular knowledge (further to that gained in pre-registration training and/or acquired only in hospital care or outside a general practice setting), it is important that items 3 and 4 in the UKCC Code of Professional Conduct are given particular consideration.

No 3 'Maintain and improve your professional knowledge and competence'.

No 4 'Acknowledge any limitations in your knowledge and competence and decline any duties or responsibilities unless able to perform them in a safe and skilled manner'.

Further information:
UKCC, 23 Portland Place, London W1N 3AF
Telephone: 071-637 7181

Indemnity for practice nurses

For practice nurses who have not taken up any indemnity, this is offered by the Royal College of Nursing or the Medical Defence Union.

The role of the practice nurse in general practice diabetes care

Nurses have been employed in general practice since 1911, but not in any number until the late 1960s following a large financial input to general practice which allowed expansion of care. In 1978 there were 3,100 and in 1984 over 6,000 nurses employed part- or whole-time in general practice, this figure increasing to over 18,000 since 1990 and changes in the National Health Service.

The role of the practice nurse has undoubtedly changed and extended with the expansion of developments in the promotion of health and the prevention and management of disease. The role encompasses four important elements in the care of the local population. These are shown in Fig 1.1.

Fig 1.1 Role of the practice nurse.

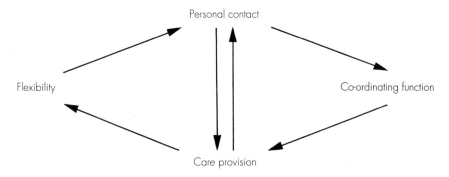

1. Personal contact

Easy and regular contact with patients is important in preventative care. Fostering good relationships with families, businesses, local services and building 'networks' takes time and entails hard work. Rewards however *are* there when a patient benefits from the results, perhaps by meeting another with a similar problem or by being put in touch with an organisation or self-help group.

Within a practice, the nurse may at times be the only health care professional on the premises when doctors are out on visits. In a large practice with many doctors and staff employed, contact with the nurse may be easier, particularly during busy surgeries or where the patient is concerned about 'bothering' the doctor.

2. Care provision

The nursing service provided in general practice allows all aspects of care of the

Fig 1.2 Nursing care provided in general practice.

	First aid/emergencies Accident prevention Immunisation Children Travel	
Health promotion Health education Disease management Health surveillance	Listen Support Advise	Treatment/procedures Screening Medicals Investigations
	Information collection Information dissemination Liaison with outside agencies	

individual and the family to be encompassed. (see Fig 1.2). These involve many activities linked by the three elements of listening, supporting and advising.

The organisation of such a workload is an important aspect of practice nursing particularly in keeping track of patients – and providing the necessary follow up care following an attendance or telephone call requesting help.

3. Co-ordinating function

The practice nurse has an important role within the practice in the education of other members of the practice team regarding raising awareness of problems, the tracking of patients, fostering good working relationships and communicating with other team members. It is in these areas in general practice, that difficulties sometimes arise, preventing the effective delivery of health care (see Fig 1.3).

The nurse's role in co-ordinating care and services 'outside' the practice is also important, particularly in relation to diabetes, where many other health care professionals and supporting services may be required in the provision of care over a person's lifetime with the condition.

4. Flexibility

Of all conditions, diabetes requires a flexible system of care from diagnosis. As far as possible – independence, choice and flexibility are 'key' factors in support, education and surveillance. In general practice, the nurse is the 'key' person to provide these elements.

Another example of flexibility encompassed by practice nurses, is the group of people with diabetes who attend neither hospital nor general practice except when they are 'ill'. This may be because they are elderly, disabled or are unaware that they require health care for their diabetes. This group may not be visited by any health care professional except in an emergency situation. The practice nurse having identified the group can take 'diabetes care' to the patient's home, arrange appropriate investigations, check that 'all is well' in the house, and if not arrange appropriate support and a follow up visit from the general practitioner at least annually.

In summary

The nurse's role in the general practice setting is a 'lynchpin' in the provision of diabetes care. His or her knowledge of the person with diabetes and the family or carers allows easy contact with the doctor or doctors (especially in a large practice) and other providers of care. Clinical care, education and record keeping are more consistent where the responsibility for these is declared and defined. Relationships built up with patients and their families encourages attendance. The success of registers, recall and follow up systems are of great importance as the basis for care outcomes and the future assessment of the practice health needs.

The nurse is in an ideal position to organise and co-ordinate a flexible service in the practice setting, where care and education can be given within surgery hours, in or out of 'protected' time, taking into account numbers, the needs of the diabetes population, the practice workload and the time of year.

Appropriately educated nurses in general practice have a very special role in the provision of care for approximately 50% of the diabetes population in the United Kingdom. In particular, in terms of organisation, patient contact, screening, recall and follow up, provision of the diabetes service with general practitioners, audit and assessment for future change and improvement in diabetes health care.

Fig 1.3 Diabetes care in general practice. Who is involved?

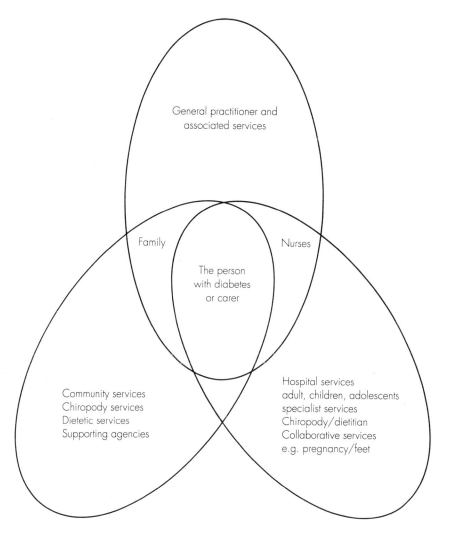

The role of receptionists, clerical staff and practice managers

Administrative staff in a practice have increasing responsibilities. Most important are those in contact every day with patients, relatives and visitors to the practice, either in person or by telephone.

Receptionists are definitely 'front line'. Their attitude, knowledge and understanding of the problems of people telephoning or attending the practice may have a bearing on whether help is sought when needed.

Clerical staff also have an important part to play in the secretarial and administrative aspects of health care – particularly where computerisation of prescriptions, information, registers and recall systems have been implemented.

In small practices there may only be a small administrative work force who know well the small practice population and very quickly can identify those with diabetes.

In a large practice or a practice with several branch surgeries, there may be many part time staff working in shifts with communications passed from one to the other in writing. It is unlikely that in this situation the 'front line' will have as much knowledge of their diabetic population.

Larger practices have for many years required the employment of a practice manager to run the business side of the practice. Fund holding practices, whether singularly or in groups, are looking at provision of care and costs associated with their practices, as well as an expanding work force. The practice manager has an increasing responsibility in these developments.

An understanding of the roles and responsibilities of administrative staff is important in diabetes care in general practice. Education of the practice manager, receptionists and clerical staff about diabetes, the treatment and acute problems requiring immediate access to the doctor or nurse enables an understanding of the problems encountered by people with diabetes and dispels some of the fear, ignorance, mystery and 'old wives' tales' surrounding this condition.

Administrative staff are in a unique position in the identification of the diabetic population with their knowledge of those attending the practice, as receivers of information and in the organisation of prescriptions. Accurate input of information regarding demography, care provision, treatment changes and other data to computer systems is vital in the audit of diabetes care and in the assessment of needs for the future.

References

British Diabetic Association Patient Services Advisory Committee (1991). *Recommendations for Diabetes Health Promotion Clinics.* British Diabetic Association, London.

General Medical Council (1987). *Professional Conduct and Discipline: Fitness to Practice*

MacKinnon, M (1990). *General Practice Diabetes Care: The Past, The Present and The Future.* Innovative Care Supplement. Diabetic Medicine 6:171-172

MacKinnon, M (1986). *Neglected Aspects in Diabetes Care: The role of nurses in General Practice.* Practical Diabetes Vol 3; No 5: 232-4

UKCC (1992). *Code of Professional Conduct for the Nurse, Midwife and Health Visitor*

2 Educational needs of the team

In a complex subject such as diabetes, an up to date knowledge and the appropriate application of knowledge is necessary for the clinical management and education of people with diabetes. Often doctors and nurses are not aware of their own continuing educational needs in order to provide the support and correct, consistent information essential for people managing their own care.

In order to ascertain educational requirements of those involved (mainly doctors and nurses), it may be helpful for members of the 'team' to identify their own learning needs by checking a 'diabetes topic' list (see Fig 2.1). This list is not inclusive of every topic, but encompasses many subjects, where clinical management, information or explanation are reliant on a level of knowledge which might be expected of the doctor or nurse, by a person with diabetes, newly diagnosed or during their diabetic life.

Fig 2.1 Diabetes knowledge – needs assessment.

Please fill in the appropriate space using the following key:

0 = No knowledge of topic
1 = Some knowledge of topic – Insufficient
2 = Good knowledge of topic – Sufficient

_____	Types of diabetes	_____	Hypos
_____	Causes of diabetes	_____	Practical aspects
_____	Inheritance	_____	Unproven methods of treatment
_____	Physiology	_____	Alternative therapy
_____	Symptoms	_____	Control
_____	Related conditions	_____	Monitoring
_____	Diet	_____	Blood glucose
_____	Overweight	_____	Urine glucose
_____	Tablets	_____	Glycosylated Hb

_____	Insulin	_____	Thrush
_____	Management (of diabetes care)	_____	HRT
_____	Brittle diabetes	_____	Termination of pregnancy
_____	Sport	_____	Infertility
_____	Eating out	_____	Genetics
_____	Holidays	_____	Pre-pregnancy
_____	Travel	_____	Pregnancy
_____	Work	_____	Gestational diabetes
_____	Other illness	_____	Baby with diabetes
_____	Sick day rules	_____	Child with diabetes
_____	Surgical operations	_____	Diabetes in adolescence
_____	Investigations	_____	A cure?
_____	Driving	_____	Complications
_____	Alcohol	_____	Feet, footwear
_____	Drugs	_____	Chiropody
_____	Smoking	_____	Retinopathy
_____	Impotence	_____	Vision
_____	Contraception	_____	Transplantation
_____	Hypertension	_____	Insulin pumps
_____	Cardiovascular problems	_____	Artificial pancreas
_____	Psychological aspects	_____	New insulins
_____	The British Diabetic Association	_____	Oral insulins
_____	Emergency treatment of hyperglycaemia	_____	Emergencies
_____	Life insurance	_____	Emergency treatment of hypoglycaemia
_____	Fructosamine	_____	Medical insurance

Members of the team may find it helpful to score themselves and note further topics of identified educational need.

_____

_____

_____

_____

_____

_____

_____

Education in diabetes – what is available for practice nurses, community nurses and general practitioners?

Mainly for nurses

Integrated or planned courses – usually based in a centre with a well developed clinical base and diabetes nurse specialist involvement.

a) *Length*
 – half day workshops
 – study days
 – 2-3 days
 – weekends
 – evenings over several weeks

b) *Evaluation* – brief to detailed questionnaires

c) *Style and content* – variable, some didactic, academic and hospital based

One off events, usually organised by a diabetes nurse specialist using 'soft' money.

Courses in academic institutions

English National Board Course No 928 in Diabetes Nursing. These are available in England. Details may be obtained from the English National Board for Nursing, Midwifery and Health Visiting (see resources list Chapter 16).

Modules on diabetes incorporated into other nursing courses for practice nurses and other nurses working in the community. These courses are validated and may lead to a practice nurse attendance certificate/diploma or community nurse qualification/diploma.

Institutions offering courses
Colleges of Nursing
Colleges of Health
Institutes of Health
Technical Colleges
Universities

Distance learning courses

Include, for example, those developed by the Manchester Diabetes Team – further details from The Manchester Diabetes Centre (see resources list Chapter 16).

Also for the whole team in general practice

Diabetes Care in General Practice – A comprehensive and interactive programme of continuing education by Dr Janet Grant and Dr Philip Marsden. Details from Eli Lilly Ltd (see resources list Chapter 16).

Other courses for nurses

- There are many developing diploma, degree and higher degree courses –
  in which diabetes may be a part or module.
- Credits or CAT points should be available on all validated courses
  where assessment is integral to the course.
- PREPP and ENB Higher Award Schemes should make continuing
  education more available for all nurses.
- District diabetes care should include in any strategy, the recognition of
  the need for local training and continuing education for nurses in
  primary care teams.
- Local or district schemes should be planned by specialist teams
  in conjunction with FHSAs and academic/continuing education institutions.

Self-help for the primary care team

- Organising own education by attending courses/conferences.
- Finding a 'buddy' practice to befriend and learn and share experiences.
- Locating a 'mentor' practice with long experience of provision of
  diabetes care.
- Contact the local diabetes team and request resources and education.
- Contact the British Diabetic Association for further information.

Mainly for general practitioners

- **Postgraduate course in diabetes held annually** – changing centres every
  two to three years. Details from specialist diabetes physicians or the British
  Diabetic Association.
- **Local initiatives** – through General Practitioner Training Schemes.
  Postgraduate Centres, RCGP Training, Diabetes Team Initiatives (PGEA
  schemes usually sought).

In summary ▬▬▬▬▬▬▬▬▬▬▬▬▬▬▬

1. Diabetes education for the primary health care team is available in some areas. Availability, accessibility and educational level, however, are variable and often reliant on 'soft' money.

2. The messages from general practice are that education is best when practice based and related to the work and development of each primary health care team. There is thus a major need for co-ordination in each district between the consumers (PHCTs), the diabetes provider teams and the education institutions and a willingness on the part of 'specialists' in diabetes to tailor their knowledge appropriately to the local community, where this is needed. Adequate funding and FHSA planning and support require further development.

Diabetes education for the primary health care team – what is needed?

Three educational units should be identified.

Unit 1 – Diabetes mellitus – an overview of the condition

Aim

To provide an opportunity for the team to obtain an overview of diabetes including the progress and treatment of the condition.

Objectives

1. Examine the physiology, aetiology and clinical picture of diabetes.
2. Discuss the epidemiology of diabetes.
3. Consider current research into diabetes and its implications in the delivery of future care.
4. Consider the available approaches for the control of blood glucose and prevention of extremes of blood glucose levels.
5. In the practice context, explore methods of screening, diagnosis and criteria for referral.
6. Examine the three modes of treatment (the food plan, medication and insulin) and their delivery in the context of age and lifestyle.

7. Identify problems of management of the control of weight, blood glucose levels and blood pressure in the ongoing care of the person with diabetes.

8. Specify the difficulties encountered by the newly diagnosed (and the family/carers) in terms of management, education and support.

9. Construct a practice guideline for the management of intercurrent illness in the person with diabetes.

10. Consider the complications of diabetes, surveillance and identification of those at risk including treatment and criteria for referral.

Unit 2 – Living with Diabetes

Aim

To enable the team to explore and understand the psychological and social implications of living with diabetes.

Objectives

1. Gain greater insight into the implications of diabetes on the lifestyle of people with diabetes and their families/carers by listening to them.

2. Develop an understanding of the problems and management in different age groups and during pregnancy.

3. Recognise the need for support and the resources available to meet this need.

4. Examine critically the role of education in diabetes care.

5. Consider the organisation and function of the hospital services, the general practice services and diabetes centres in the delivery of care.

6. Identify the role of other health care professionals in diabetes care and the pathways of referral to them.

7. Explore the important role of voluntary organisations in diabetes care, in particular the role of the British Diabetic Association.

Unit 3 – The management of diabetes care in general practice

Aim

To provide an opportunity for the primary health care team to examine their own practice management of diabetes care.

Objectives

1. Identify the aims and objectives of the practice diabetes service.

2. Discuss the purpose of the diabetes service in general practice.

3. Specify the skills required to run the service.

4. Analyse the organisation required.

5. Describe methods of evaluation and audit of the service.

6. Consider the identification and systems for registration, follow up and recall of people with diabetes in the practice.

7. Design realistic and effective educational aims and objectives applicable to the practice diabetes population.

8. Construct protocols for:

    a) Initial assessment of newly diagnosed patients

    b) A routine review

    c) An annual review

9. List short and long term aims for the practice diabetes service.

10. Explore methods of 'team work' in terms of working together and problem solving.

Reference

Roberts, S; MacKinnon, M; Braid, E (1992) *Draft Report on Educational Initiatives in Diabetes for General Practitioners and their teams.* Unpublished Report. British Diabetic Association, Education Section.

3 Diabetes mellitus in the United Kingdom

Prevalence and incidence

There are estimated to be between 500,000 and 750,000 people with clinically diagnosed diabetes in the United Kingdom (see Fig 3.1). These figures suggest that the combined prevalence of insulin dependent diabetes and non-insulin dependent diabetes is just over 1% of the white British population. Undiagnosed people with diabetes brings the total to 1 million or more. The prevalence of diabetes is considerably higher in the older age groups and, over the age of 65 years, over 4% of the population has diabetes. Over the age of 75 years this figure may increase to as much as 10% of the population.

Fig 3.1 The prevalence of diabetes in the UK population in relation to age.

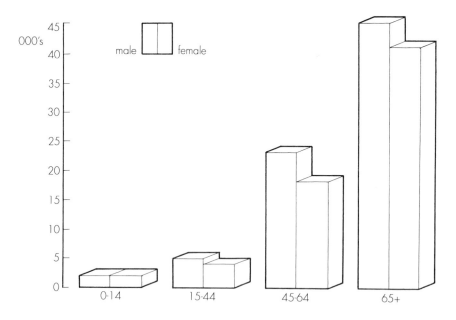

(British Diabetic Association Report 1988. Diabetes in the United Kingdom)

Figures available for the prevalence of diabetes in children and young people (under the age of 11 years) show that this condition has become more common over the last 20 years and that the increase is mainly in social classes I and II. The prevalence of insulin dependent diabetes in people under the age of 20 years is 1.22 per 1,000 which means that there are probably more than 18,000 young people with diabetes in the United Kingdom.

People with non-insulin dependent diabetes may remain undiagnosed for months or years. The condition may only be diagnosed by coincidence, following routine screening (eg at a medical examination, a routine out-patient visit or prior to surgery).

The number of new cases of diabetes diagnosed each year in the United Kingdom is estimated to be 60,000 (British Diabetic Association).

Racial variations

High rates of diabetes are found in the Asian population in the United Kingdom. The prevalence is approximately four times higher than that found in the white population. The prevalence of diabetes in Asians is further increased with age, to as much as 16% in the 40-65 age range – four to five times higher than the white population of similar age.

Afro-Caribbean people in the United Kingdom also have a slightly higher prevalence of non-insulin dependent diabetes, associated with weight gain.

Both these populations are more at risk of cardiac disease, a significant complication of diabetes.

The complications of diabetes

Retinopathy

Surveys show that 30% of all people with diabetes have retinopathy and about 1%-2% develop sight threatening changes each year. If these are detected early enough, usually before vision is affected, laser treatment will prevent 70% from going blind. In 1980, diabetes was the most common cause of blindness in people aged 45-64 years. People with diabetes in that age group were 23 times more likely to be blind than their non-diabetic contemporaries. Over 65 years, they are twice as likely to be blind.

Nephropathy

A survey in 1985 found that 580 people with diabetes in the United Kingdom developed renal failure. About 450 were thought suitable for treatment, but it was only possible to provide dialysis or transplantation for about 270 of them.

Neuropathy

Evidence of neuropathy may be found in as many as 60% of people with diabetes, causing problems for about one third of them. One of the most distressing and often hidden problems is that of male impotence.

Foot ulceration

Foot ulceration is at least 50 times more common in people with diabetes than in the non-diabetic population. If the ulceration is due to peripheral vascular disease, amputation is often the outcome. Over the age of 65 years, people with diabetes are 25 times more likely to have had a leg amputated than those without diabetes. Collaborative foot clinics have shown that with a specialist team approach the need for amputation can be halved.

The consequences of diabetes

- **Mortality**

- **Heart attacks**

- **Strokes**

- **Kidney failure**

- **Peripheral vascular disease**

- **Diabetic ketosis**

Mortality

It is recognised that people with diabetes die earlier than those of a similar age and sex without the condition. Death may be directly due to diabetes (eg diabetic ketoacidosis or renal failure due to diabetes). More commonly, however, death is due to macrovascular complications, particularly myocardial infarctions and strokes.

It is suggested that approximately 40,000 people with diabetes die each year in the United Kingdom. If analysed by age and sex, it seems that about 20,000 die prematurely each year as the result of having diabetes. Premature deaths are more marked in women than in men and more obvious in the younger age groups. Deaths occur due to heart attacks, strokes and peripheral vascular disease.

A study of death in 448 people with diabetes from various parts of the United Kingdom under the age of 50 years was carried out in 1979. In this survey, the two commonest causes of death of people with diabetes under the age of 50 were heart attacks and kidney failure.

Heart attacks

Overall, people with diabetes are more likely to die of heart attacks than people without diabetes. In men it is 1.9 times more common than in non-diabetics – in women the figure is 2.7 times higher. In younger patients (under 45) the increased risk of dying from a heart attack is much greater, five times more likely in men and 11.5 times more likely in women.

Strokes

Women with diabetes are twice as likely to die from strokes, men about 1.5 times more likely. There is an increased risk of mortality from strokes in younger people with diabetes.

Kidney failure

This is a common cause of death in those who develop diabetes before they are 30 years old. In a survey of people dying from kidney failure before 50 years of age, death was found to be 40 times more common in people with diabetes. Recent surveys however, have shown that as treatment has improved over the last 40 years, the incidence of nephropathy and kidney failure has decreased by about one third. Renal failure can now be treated by dialysis or renal transplantation.

Peripheral vascular disease

Although the number of deaths among people with diabetes from this cause is not so high, there are about 2.5 times more deaths than would be expected in non-diabetics of the same age and sex.

Diabetic ketosis

In the 1979 survey carried out by the BDA and RCP, 74 of the 448 people with diabetes studied died from diabetic ketosis. If this condition does develop, early treatment should lead to the condition being corrected. Death in these patients was often due to psychological problems and delays in treatment.

The cost of diabetes

In the United Kingdom people with diabetes consume between 4% and 5% of health care resources. The cost of diabetes to the NHS during 1989 is estimated to have been £1 billion. Patients with diabetes have a hospital bed occupancy of about double that for all other categories of patients combined.

Direct costs to the NHS include in-patient and out-patient care provided by hospitals, services provided by general practitioners and district nurses in the community and the cost of supplies – insulin, tablets, syringes, needle clippers and monitoring strips. In addition, there are costs involved, particularly in screening for and treating retinopathy, in the treatment of end stage renal failure and the specials costs incurred by those who have suffered amputation.

Indirect costs to the individual of unfulfilled ambitions, the psychological effect of combined anxieties about living with diabetes and the prospect of developing complications cannot be quantified. The costs of loss of earning capacity resulting from ill health or premature death are unknown, although estimated to be significant compared to the non-diabetic population.

Good evidence is available that regional costs could be reduced by a number of inexpensive measures. For example:

1. The provision of sufficient interested and trained physicians and nurses working with dietitians and chiropodists.
2. Adequate education facilities for people with diabetes and their families.
3. Resources and support for general practitioners and their teams caring for the non-hospital diabetic population.

Effectiveness of treatment for people with diabetes

The maintenance of near physiological blood glucose levels is believed to reduce the risk of development of long term complications. Early detection and treatment of established complications can reduce morbidity and costs.

For example, in retinopathy, the detection of early changes, followed by laser treatment, can prevent blindness. Planned follow up with screening for complications is essential. Living with diabetes involves lifestyle modification to achieve optimal control of the condition. Time spent in listening, responding to questions and providing information and support is as essential to treatment as the prescription of diet, diet and medication, or diet and insulin.

In summary

1. Diabetes is a common condition.

2. With modern methods of treatment, people with diabetes can look forward to a near normal life.

3. If treatment is less than optimal, acute illness may necessitate hospital admission. Complications affecting the eyes, kidneys and feet may seriously affect the quality of life.

4. Diabetes can be costly to the patient and the NHS. Properly planned services and preventive activities can greatly reduce the cost to both.

5. Present treatment of diabetes does not only depend on technology. An important aspect of care is the education of the patient and family.

The aims of diabetes care

The overall aims of any system of diabetes care are to facilitate diabetic self-management and control, enabling people with diabetes to make the necessary adjustments to remain well and happy, to reduce mortality, morbidity and hospitalisation and to improve the early detection of complications by effective surveillance.

How is diabetes care organised in the United Kingdom?

There continues to be considerable variation in the standard of care provided for people with diabetes. Most districts have specialist diabetes clinics although these vary in quality. In some districts people with diabetes are followed up in general medical clinics. Increasingly, hospital clinics are being set up collaboratively for special problems. There may be joint clinics with obstetricians, joint renal clinics and foot clinics including the expertise of vascular surgeons, chiropodists and orthotists (fitters of shoes and other applicances).

In many districts, clinics for children with diabetes are organised, run by a paediatrician with a special interest in diabetes. Out of hours peripheral clinics are available in some areas, providing a service for the adolescent and working populations.

Approximately half the diabetic population regularly attends a hospital clinic with the specialist facilities this provides. Those attending the hospital are mainly the younger population (treated with diet and insulin) and those with established complications requiring particular surveillance and treatment.

The remaining 50% of the diabetic population are either cared for by their general practitioner and team or they receive no care at all. At the present time (1993), it is estimated that approximately 50% of general practices in the United Kingdom are providing an organised service of diabetes care. The remaining 50% of practices provide little or no care for their diabetic population.

Mainly, interested general practitioners and their teams are looking after the non-insulin dependent diabetic population, where diabetes occurs in middle and later life. Often this type of diabetes has been regarded as mild. This is not so. Non-insulin dependent diabetes affects 75% of the diabetic population; it is associated with all the complications of diabetes, which are not uncommonly already present at diagnosis.

The organisation of diabetes care is complex and ever-changing in the life of a person with diabetes, not only from the person's own perspective but also in the multitude of relatives and professionals who may be involved in his/her care, individually or collectively.

Support, education, good communications and an understanding of the availability of appropriate care by the person with diabetes, relatives and health care professionals are as important as the treatment of the condition.

The role of the specialist team

The specialist team in diabetes care has evolved over a number of years. The team includes

- Physician/paediatrician
- Nurse specialist
- Dietitian
- Chiropodist

The team may be extended under certain circumstances to include:

- Obstetrician
- Vascular surgeon
- Ophthalmologist
- Renal physician
- Psychologist

The team should provide the expertise (based on training and experience) for the management of care of diabetes in the hospital setting and be available as a resource for care in the community.

The physician (diabetologist)
- Has a specialist *interest, training* and *experience* in the management of diabetes.
- May have *research* interests.
- Is involved in the *leadership* of diabetes care in a district.
- Should be a *resource* for medical practitioners and health care professionals.
- Is dedicated to *raising awareness* of diabetes.
- Competes for *finance* and *resources* to support diabetes.

It is important that general practitioners and their teams providing diabetes care are aware of the physician(s) with a specialist interest in the district. Should problems arise, they will be quickly resolved where links have been established and communication is easy.

Many centres also have a paediatrician with a particular interest and training in the care of children and young people with diabetes. The paediatrician's team will consist of a nurse specialist (sometimes children-trained) and a dietitian specialising in the needs of children.

Ideally, as children move towards adulthood, a collaborative service should be available where the paediatrician and physician caring for adults work together with appropriate teams to ensure that the change from childhood care to adult care is as smooth as possible.

The nurse specialist
The nurse specialist is a trained nurse with extended knowledge and skills in diabetes management as an educator, manager, researcher, communicator and innovator held responsible for his or her actions.

Diabetes nurse specialists work wholly in diabetes care, either full- or part-time with a physician(s) or paediatrician(s) involved in diabetes. The nurse may be based in hospital or community but may visit in either depending on need. The nurse works either with adults or children with diabetes and their families, or with both. The nurse is a resource and advisor in diabetes for other health professionals in the health authority. The nurse specialist is an educator of colleagues in nursing and other disciplines in hospital and community and, working within the diabetes care team, provides the following services:

- A newly diagnosed person – help for the whole family in understanding and coming to terms with the condition.
- Stabilisation of people new to insulin.
- Understanding blood sugar control and how to monitor this. Advice on monitoring systems.
- Prevention of hypoglycaemia.
- Advice in the prevention and treatment of hyperglycaemia (eg during illness).

- Changing insulin regimes or insulin injections systems.
- Understanding and knowledge of diabetic complications.
- Prevention of foot problems.
- Education on all aspects of diabetes, individually or in groups for people with diabetes and colleagues.
- Support for the person with diabetes, the family and carers.
- Crisis management – in particular where there are psychological, social and family problems.
- Facilitating all aspects of diabetes care with appropriate health care professionals and others (eg teachers, employers).
- Providing the necessary expertise and materials or resources where requested or required.

Nurse specialists have incorporated into their job description the necessary authorisation for the alteration of insulin and medication in the treatment of diabetes. This authorisation is only provided with the agreement of the diabetologist or physician involved and following training in the management of diabetes by the nurse specialist. In addition many nurse specialists provide an out of hours, weekend advisory service. It is well recognised that this is valued by people with diabetes, particularly by the newly diagnosed person/child or their family/carers. A telephone call for advice may prevent an emergency situation arising.

The dietitian
The particular responsibilities of the dietitian in diabetes care include:

- Assessment of eating habits (individual and family).
- Advice on buying and cooking food.
- Ensuring adequate nutrition (especially in the young, elderly).
- Promoting healthy eating.
- Helping people to reduce weight.
- Stabilising weight.
- Meal planning (especially regular meals).
- Advice and planning of special dietary needs (eg for people in renal failure).

Interested dietitians are often involved in all aspects of diabetes support and education, either to individuals or groups. However, they may also be involved in the provision of other dietetic services. In general, dietitians are hospital based, working with their colleagues and linking in with the diabetologist and nurse specialist.

Community dietitians are spread thinly in the United Kingdom. Some districts do have them and they can be a valuable resource for dietetic advice in the community, in particular to general practice. In many districts, however, where no community dietitian is available, the person with diabetes is provided with dietetic advice by the practice nurse, district nurse, health visitor or general practitioner – often with very little training in the specific aspects of diabetic dietary requirements. It is the right of every person with diabetes to receive advice from a trained dietitian, who may be hospital based, and is available in every district.

The dietitian should be an important resource in the provision of training and continuing education of all those providing diabetes care in the community. More community dietitians are required to meet this need.

The chiropodist

Within the NHS, each district provides a chiropody service in community clinics and hospitals and at home for housebound patients. Referrals come from doctors, nurses or patients themselves. Some hospitals and general practices provide chiropody within their diabetic clinics. The NHS employs only State Registered Chiropodists (SRCh) who have trained for three years at one of the recognised schools. State Registered Chiropodists also practise privately, as do unregistered chiropodists with varying amounts of training. Care should be taken therefore when referring people to a private chiropodist. Podiatrists are chiropodists with extended training.

Chiropody services for people with diabetes

Both neuropathic and ischaemic ulcers are commonest in diabetic patients. The chiropodist has an important role in the teaching of all aspects of foot care. This includes advice about nail cutting and shoes to avoid the development of foot ulcers and in managing existing ulcers. A specialised multi-disciplinary foot clinic can halve the number of amputations in diabetic patients as long as referral to these clinics is appropriate and in good time.

Most health authorities expect chiropodists to provide services for patients in four official priority groups:

• Old age pensioners
• Children attending school
• Mentally or physically handicapped
• Pregnant women

Surprisingly, people with diabetes are not officially recognised as a priority group, but many chiropody services do accept referrals of people with diabetes and other high risk groups. At present most District Health Authorities do not purchase chiropody for otherwise well people between the ages of 16 and 65 years. Ideally, a range of foot problems should be officially recognised in the

NHS. A more coherent policy is required, based on unmet need and its associated morbidity.

Chiropodists with an up to date knowledge of diabetes care have an important role in the prevention of disability in the management of diabetic foot problems. Their expertise includes:

- Assessment of foot structure and function
- The manufacture of orthoses (insoles, padding, special shoes)
- Advice on shoes/shoe fitting
- Ongoing surveillance
- Treatment (eg reduction of callus, nail care, debriding of ulcers).

A list of State Registered Chiropodists employed by the health authority is available in every district, in headquarters or community units. Lists of private State Registered Chiropodists are available in *Yellow Pages*. Fees for private chiropody services vary. Home visits are more costly than visits to a surgery.

Diabetes centres
Education of the person with diabetes and the family is a key factor in the reduction of morbidity, mortality and the need for hospital admission. Improved education programmes may not only reduce the number of foot complications, but also drastically reduce admission rates for hypoglycaemia, ketoacidosis and the demands on accident and emergency departments as well as achieving improvement in overall blood glucose control.

A hospital clinic is not the place for education programmes. Clinics may be large, busy and often staffed by inexperienced and frequently changing junior doctors. In an out-patient clinic there are major obstacles to the success of education programmes, where time and skilled counselling may not be available and where the clinic environment is inappropriate.

The purpose of diabetes centres
There are many diabetes centres in the United Kingdom and more are planned.

The diabetes centre is a base for the specialist team and a focus for care provision and resources within the district. Its functions include provision of

1. A register of all patients in the district in order to support hospital-based and general practitioner care systems and ensure adequate supervision or follow up.

2. Appropriate organisation and a pleasant environment for effective patient education (individually or in groups) which ensures the development and achievement of agreed objectives with

- Primary education programmes for people with newly diagnosed diabetes (and their families/carers).
- Secondary education: long term diabetes control counselling and maintenance and re-enforcement of changes in behaviour.

3. A communication centre to
- Provide a reference point for patient enquiries.
- Ensure co-ordination between members of the diabetes team enabling the formulation and implementation of agreed objectives.
- Provide integration with other hospital departments and staff to achieve common treatment policies.
- Help general practitioner co-operative care schemes achieve common goals.
- Act as a focal point for the training of medical and non-medical staff.
- Streamline organisation and improve cost-effectiveness.

4. A comprehensive system of clinical care and evaluation should ensure
- Out-patient care of all new and follow up patients.
- Effective screening and surveillance procedures for complications.
- Availability of facilities for treatment of diabetic complications and referral for non-diabetic medical problems.
- The development, maintenance and support of general practitioner co-operative care schemes.

The British Diabetic Association

The role of the British Diabetic Association in the organisation of diabetes care in the United Kingdom

The British Diabetic Association (founded in 1934) has 140,000 members, mainly people with diabetes, those who care for them and health professionals, all with the common goal of improving care and quality of life for those with diabetes. Professional membership is organised into the Medical and Scientific section, and Education and Professional Care section. All meet regularly to exchange new information and ideas. Many clinicians with a special concern for diabetes are members and as a group have collected considerable data on many aspects of diabetes.

The BDA also funds diabetes research. Of particular relevance is a current research project, the UK Prospective Diabetes Study, funded by the MRTC, BDA and the pharmaceutical industry, which addresses the complication rates in non-insulin dependent diabetes (NIDDM). This study has been in progress for over 10 years and should give important answers as to the best available treatment for NIDDM by 1995.

The Association has an important role in any countrywide strategy for raising health care standards in the United Kingdom.

The BDA provides an authoritative source of information on living with diabetes to people with diabetes, those who care for them and health professionals. Activities include organising and contributing to scientific meetings and training courses, producing leaflets on specific topics and other educational material and programmes for children and young people with diabetes. Information covers treatment, lifestyle, care and social aspects of diabetes. The Association's magazine *Balance* (readership around 250,000) is an important medium of communication countrywide. *Balance for Beginners* (for IDDM and NIDDM) is an important resource for those newly diagnosed with diabetes or for people wanting an update. This is freely available on request to general practice clinics and individuals with diabetes/carers. Contact the British Diabetic Association (see resources list Chapter 16).

The BDA has three main departments under the Services Division. These are:
- Diabetes care
- Diet information
- Youth department

1. Diabetes care
This department deals with any questions relating to diabetes care from people with diabetes or health care professionals on any topic (eg insurance, driving, travel, benefits, aspects of care).

2. Diet information
Two qualified dietitians and a home economist are available, providing dietary advice and suggestions regarding healthy eating and meal planning as well as creating recipes. These are available in published form. To order – telephone or write for a free catalogue.

3. Youth department
The Youth department provides services for children and young people with diabetes from the onset of their diabetes to the age of 25 years (and for anyone else involved with them: parents, teachers, careers officers and others). They run holiday and activity courses throughout the United Kingdom for children aged 5-18. Family weekends are run from October to April. Youth packs and school packs are also provided by this department.

BDA branches

There are over 400 local branches of the BDA across Britain and Northern Ireland. They are all run by volunteers with support from the local area co-ordinator, also a volunteer. A contact list is available comprising: parent groups (young people with diabetes), youth diabetes groups, self-help groups, Asian support groups, groups for the visually impaired as well as ordinary branches who have regular meetings. The whole of this voluntary section is co-ordinated at its Queen Anne Street headquarters in London, where information can be obtained regarding local groups, through the Liaison Officer.

Funding of the British Diabetic Association

The BDA is funded entirely by voluntary contributions. No government funding is provided to support the organisation. One particular countrywide event which takes place every year during June is National Diabetes Week. During this week, local branch members are involved in house-to-house collections, and can be seen in high streets.

The British Diabetic Association is an important non-government organisation dedicated to raising awareness of diabetes and in attracting funds in order to support diabetes and research in the United Kingdom.

The British Diabetic Association and general practice

It has been recognised by the association that there has been a rapid expansion of diabetes care provided in general practice. Several initiatives are in place for the support of general practitioners and their teams.

* A working group for general practice diabetes care.
* Resources for general practitioners and their teams (information packs, leaflets, books).
* Opportunities to share information and learn in conferences and study days.
* Information on courses in diabetes.
* Encouragement of practices to join the BDA to obtain regular up to date information.
* Specialist services available.
* Services of the Information Department.

The Information Department

The Information Department provides a database for health care professionals providing bibliographies and a bi-monthly list of all relevant publications. Contact the British Diabetic Association (see resources list Chapter 16).

References

British Diabetic Association. *Balance.* Issued bi-monthly.

British Diabetic Association. *Insulin Dependent Diabetes Balance for Beginners.* Updated annually.

British Diabetic Association. *Non-Insulin Dependent Diabetes Balance for Beginners.* Updated annually.

British Diabetic Association (1988). *Diabetes in the United Kingdom.* British Diabetic Association, London.

Consumers Association (1991). *What Chiropody Offers.* Drug and Therapeutics Bulletin Vol 29; No 8: 29-30

Day J L; Spathis M (1988). *District Diabetes Centres in the United Kingdom.* Workshop Report. Diabetic Medicine 5: 372-380.

Joint Working Party on Diabetic Renal Failure of the British Diabetic Association, The Renal Association and The Research Unit of the Royal College of Physicians (1988). *Renal failure in diabetes in the UK: deficient provision of care in 1985.* Diabetic Medicine 5: 79-84

Murphy M (1991). *The Health of the Nation. Response from the British Diabetic Association.* British Diabetic Association, London.

Royal College of Nursing Diabetes Nursing Forum Document (1991). *The Role of the Specialist Nurse.* Royal College of Nursing.

Tunbridge WMG (1981). *Factors contributing to deaths of diabetics under fifty years of age .* The Lancet 2: 569-572

Watkins P J; Drury P L; Taylor K W (1990). *Diabetes and its Management.* Blackwell Scientific Publications.

Part 2 Providing diabetes care

4 The diabetes service in general practice

How to set up a system of care

Aims

1. To identify, know and register the diabetes population covered by the practice.

2. To provide treatment, support, education and surveillance for people with diabetes not receiving hospital care or where care is 'shared'. (For definition of 'shared care' for people with diabetes see page 38).

3. To know and use all available specialist and support services – referring to these in good time and appropriately.

Objectives

1. Planning and organisation of registration, recall and follow up systems and their regular update.

2. A planned programme of care for all those receiving the practice diabetes service including:

a) Initial support, assessment and treatment of newly diagnosed people with diabetes including immediate referral for specialist services, where appropriate.

b) Initial and staged continuing education that is correct, consistent and up to date.

c) Planned appropriate treatment (taking into account age, lifestyle, knowledge and understanding), that achieves the maintenance of near normal blood glucose control.

d) Management of acute complications (such as hyperglycaemia, ketosis and hypoglycaemia).

e) Identification of risk factors for long term effects of diabetes, such as:

   i Hypertension

   ii Hyperlipidaemia

f) Early identification, surveillance, treatment (and referral, if appropriate) of long term complications of diabetes in order to reduce:

   i Blindness and visual impairment

   ii Foot ulceration, limb amputation disability

   iii End stage renal failure

   iv Premature ill health and early death resulting from the macrovascular complications of ischaemic heart disease, peripheral vascular disease and cerebrovascular disease

Planning the service

Careful planning by the practice team will involve:

1. Knowledge of the practice diabetes population in terms of numbers, type of diabetes (treatment) and who is currently providing their care.

2. Organisation of the service (in relation to other services provided by the practice).

3. Availability of the necessary skills.

4. Identification of training or continuing education requirements by members of the team involved.

5. Necessary equipment, education material and resources required (other than those currently available in the practice).

6. Methods of record keeping to be employed.

7. Planning the start date for the service in relation to the necessary preparation period.

   Involvement and discussion by members of the team will identify possible organisational problems and resource implications early.

   It may be helpful for a member of the local hospital specialist team or specialist facilitator to be invited to the practice during the planning period. This would have the advantages of:

a) Establishing a relationship and communication between the practice and the hospital diabetes team.

b) Signifying the practice's intentions and plans for their service so that the specialist team are aware of them.

c) Providing awareness of the available local and national diabetes specialist and support facilities.

d) Setting up the necessary links for sharing care.

e) Discussion around diabetes management and local protocols for care, criteria for referral and mechanisms for urgent referral (such as a newly diagnosed child with diabetes or a person with foot ulceration).

f) Training or updating requirements by the team to be involved in the practice diabetes service.

Planning the service will also involve consideration of dietetic, chiropody and perhaps counselling services. Depending on district services available, the practice may decide to provide these 'in house'.

It is important that if expertise is acquired by the practice in these areas, that the professionals employed are qualified (ie State Registered Dietitians and State Registered Chiropodists) and that they have an up to date knowledge of current diabetes management.

The planning period should also encompass plans for the ongoing review of the diabetes service and consideration of its evaluation and annual audit. It is also a useful time for discussion with local services (such as pharmacists, opticians) to raise awareness regarding the proposed diabetes service.

Finally, and most important, the preparation time before the commencement of the service should include discussion about diabetes, identifying any problems that members of the team may have in the future provision of a high quality service for people with diabetes in the care of the practice.

Organisation of the service

Practices vary in their organisation of diabetes care, often the system employed relates to the size of practice.

Small practices with one general practitioner may only have 20 people identified with diabetes. If a third or a half of these receive care provided by the hospital services, the number cared for in the practice is small, perhaps not warranting even a monthly clinic. Such a practice may provide a service to individuals within surgery time. Some general practitioners may prefer this, so long as there is an established recall system and there is enough time during the consultation to provide an adequate service. In larger practices, a regular 'diabetes' clinic may be required within protected time.

The advantage of 'protected' time in a diabetes clinic is that the focus at that time is on diabetes care. People with diabetes attending the practice are aware that the diabetes clinic is on a certain day at the same time and regular attendance becomes routine. However, it is important that people unable to attend such a 'clinic' because of work or other commitments can be offered the service at other times. Organising a service that is flexible also encourages attendance.

Another group who need to be identified are people with diabetes who are housebound and unable to attend the surgery, and not receiving diabetes care and surveillance from the hospital or any other health care provider. District nurses are involved in diabetes care for those who are dependent for their care in the short or long term. The care provided by district nurses is usually related to treatment – the administration of insulin, foot/leg dressings or supervision of these, and monitoring diabetes control. Management of diabetes and surveillance for problems and detection of complications in the housebound will need inclusion in the organisation of the practice service by the team involved. The district nurse or practice nurse should visit the housebound regularly, discussing care with the general practitioner who will provide a follow up visit periodically and at least an annual review.

Who might be offered the practice diabetes service?

In every district, it is to be hoped that discussions will have been held between specialist teams and general practitioners as to the arrangements for diabetes care provision and suggested criteria for referral and sharing care.

The service could be offered to:

1. People with non-insulin dependent diabetes.
2. Some people with insulin dependent diabetes.
3. People with diabetes *wishing* to attend the practice for their care.
4. Those who are very elderly or frail for whom hospital care is inappropriate unless absolutely essential.
5. Those who are housebound.
6. Those discharged from hospital care or where no care provision is identified.
7. Those attending hospital for *other* conditions, where diabetes care, education and surveillance are not provided by *other* specialists.

Who will be involved in the provision of the practice diabetes service?

A minimum team, in a moderate to large practice, would consist of a reception-ist/secretary, nurse and doctor. In a large practice more than one receptionist/secretary and nurse may be required to keep the service and its administration running throughout the year. In a practice where many doctors may be in partnership, which doctor or doctors will be involved requires clarifi-cation at an early stage. In some practices all the medical practitioners wish to be involved in the total care of their own patients. This system is feasible, so long as the person running the service (eg the nurse) communicates with each doctor about the care of each patient. The argument put forward in favour of this system is that all the medical practitioners retain their skill in the manage-ment of diabetes.

However, a disadvantage of this system is that all the doctors may not be able to retain their knowledge and skills with very few patients to manage. It is therefore probably best, in the interests of a quality service, for one doctor in the practice to take overall responsibility for diabetes care. Continuing education and the management of many patients will ensure retention of knowledge and skills. This doctor can provide the necessary leadership for the diabetes service, at the same time communicating with colleagues about the service and the progress of their individual patients. Further, the identified team will provide continuity and consistency of information – important in diabetes care where conflicting messages are often received by people with diabetes in their dealings with many health care professionals.

The nurse's role is also important in continuity of care, in the support and education of clerks and reception staff and in communicating with the doctors in the practice and other providers of care.

Provision of the service – day, time and frequency

In order to decide on the best day, time and how often the service will be provided, the following should be considered:

1. Numbers of people with diabetes (see page 38).
2. Those requiring practice diabetes care.
3. Those requiring shared care (see page 38).
4. Organisation for patients usually attending a branch surgery (perhaps more than one, especially in rural areas).
5. Primary health services already offered by the practice.
6. Availability of medical, nursing and administration time.
7. Appropriate and available facilities (rooms, storage of equipment, educational materials).
8. Transport services, especially for those visually impaired or disabled.
9. Organisation for annual review, where eye screening may be arranged as a separate session(s) annually.
10. Availability and timing of laboratory collections (eg venous blood taken for measurement of glycosylated haemoglobin should be collected the same day or stored in the refrigerator and collected no later than the next day).
11. Sufficient time for individual patient care and education at a routine appointment (at least 20 minutes) and at annual review (at least 30 minutes). More time may be required.
12. Identified time within the clinic for administration, record keeping and individual follow up care that may be required for individual patients (eg arranging for chiropody, obtaining advice from a diabetes team, enquiring about appropriate social services benefits).
13. Extra time or 'leeway' of time should be available for:
   a) New patients to the practice.
   b) People with newly diagnosed diabetes.
   c) Those with diabetes requiring urgent care or advice for a specific problem which cannot or should not be left until the next scheduled appointment.

Numbers of people with diabetes

In a large practice where numbers may be high (perhaps due to an older population) or the ethnic composition is high (eg Asian, Afro-Caribbean), it may be necessary to hold a clinic every week. In a small practice, a clinic may only be required monthly or even bi-monthly.

Shared care

In the management of diabetes, the provision of care should aim to be organised and individual to the person concerned. During the lifetime of a person with diabetes, care is provided by the primary care team or a specialist team, or both. The appropriate care provider will change according to the progress of the condition, the need for optimum management and the wishes of the person with diabetes.

Where care is 'shared' it is important that each provider is aware of the other in the diabetes management and that the person with diabetes understands the nature of the care provided by primary care and specialist teams.

In 'shared' care good communication and record keeping are essential by all providers. A person care card (co-operation card) held by the person with diabetes may be useful so long as it is filled in by those concerned! Care provision (who does what, where and when) is an important part of diabetes education for all people with diabetes.

Finally, it is important that 'shared' care is understood by all concerned – *with* each individual person with diabetes. Where these demarcations do not exist, care may be duplicated or not provided at all.

Ideal facilities for the diabetes service

There are no special facilities necessary for diabetes care other than those that would be provided for all primary health care.

Consideration should be given to flexible use of the waiting area, perhaps for periodic educational group sessions when discussions can be held and videos shown. This area may also be used for the display of literature about diabetes and information regarding local services and facilities along with other health care educational material.

No particular clinical room facilities are necessary, other than a dark room, where fundoscopy examination will take place, and space for the correct distance to be measured between the patient and the Snellen Chart (for testing vision). A six metre distance and chart are commonly used, although in a small surgery a three metre chart can be obtained or a six metre chart used with a mirror (see section on testing for visual acuity in Chapter 11).

Who does what in which room is often a cause for debate! Where the nurse and doctor are setting up a new service, it may be helpful for both to work together in one room until confidence is gained and each understands the other's role. Later, the organisation may change to clinical checks and education provided by the nurse, a review of these by the doctor with further medical checks, discussion and prescription to complete the periodic or annual review and the follow up care decided appropriately.

It should be remembered that people with diabetes attending the surgery or medical centre may be elderly, visually impaired or disabled and any facilities for diabetes care should accommodate these problems.

Essential equipment

General

1. Hand washing facilities with warm water, soap and paper towels –
Important for finger prick tests for blood glucose levels and good hygiene.

2. **Weighing scales (metric or imperial)** –
These should be checked and calibrated annually.

3. **Weight conversion chart (kilos-stones/pounds)** –
Available from visiting pharmaceutical representatives.

4. **'Ideal' weight chart** –
ie weight for height of men and women (available from pharmaceutical representatives.)

5. **Height gauge** – correctly positioned.

6. **Equipment for collection of laboratory samples** –
eg blood, urine, wound swabs.

7. **Sphygmomanometer** with standard cuff
– small and large cuffs should also be available and these should be checked annually. (3M Health Care Ltd provides a FREE service – see resources list Chapter 16).

8. **Disposable gloves**

9. **Sharps disposal container**

Screening and monitoring

Note
Multiple urine test strips are available, though expensive (Boehringer Mannheim and Ames).

1. **Clock or wrist watch with second hand** – Essential for the correct timing of urine and capillary blood tests.

2. **White cotton wool/tissues for removal of blood from test strips** – Coloured cotton wool/tissues should not be used as they may affects results.

Screening

1. **For glucose and protein in the urine** – Strips such as Uristix (Ames) are required as well as measurement of blood glucose if glycosuria is found. Occasionally an oral glucose tolerance test (OGTT) is necessary (see section *Screening for diabetes mellitus* in Chapter 5).

2. **Lucozade 375 ml or 75 g glucose for OGTT** – Glucose may be obtained on prescription if the patient is exempt from charges, otherwise it is cheaper (than paying a prescription charge) to buy ready measured from the pharmacy (see section *Oral glucose tolerance test* in Chapter 5).

Monitoring

Urine testing
1. **For glucose in the urine (quantitative)** – Diastix (Ames) or Diabur Test 5000 (Boehringer Mannheim).
Note Ketones may inhibit colour change in Diastix.

2. **For protein in the urine (quantitative)** – Albustix (Ames) or Albym (Boehringer Mannheim).

3. **For microalbuminuria** – Micral Test (Boehringer Mannheim – strips) or Nyocard-U-Albumin (Nycomed UK Limited – tablets).

4. **For ketones in the urine** – Ketostix (Ames) or Ketur Test (Boehringer Mannheim). For use in illness (and on diagnosis).

Capillary blood testing
1. **Finger pricking devices/lancets for multiple use** – Soft Touch (Boehringer Mannheim); Unistik; Autolet (Owen Mumford); Glucolet; Glucolet II (Ames).

Note Lancets are available on FP10. Finger pricking devices can be purchased or available via hospital prescription.

2. **Test strips for blood glucose measurement** – BM-Test 1-44 Sticks (Boehringer Mannheim) or Glucostix (Ames). Both available on FP10.

3. **Blood glucose meters and test strips appropriate to the meter used.**
Note Meters are *not* essential (even though they may be given away free). If the practice is given or purchases a meter, care should be taken to calibrate it with the correct strips and quality control solution used to monitor the accuracy of the instrument.

Testing for peripheral neuropathy
1. **Patella hammer** – for checking reflexes.

2. **Tuning fork** – for checking vibration sensation (CO 128).

3. **Cotton wool/pin** – for checking lower limb sensation.

Checking visual acuity
1. **Snellen chart** – well lit.

2. **Tape** – to mark distance on floor for patient to view chart.

3. **Pinhole card** – to be held in front of the eye by the patient to discount errors of refraction, should visual acuity be reduced.

Fundoscopy – screening for diabetic retinopathy
1. **Ophthalmoscope** – with spare bulb and charged batteries (regular checking required).

2. **Mydriatic drops** – for dilating pupils, eg Tropicamide 5%.

For emergency use – for the treatment of hypoglycaemia
In surgery
Lucozade/glucose tablets
Hypostop gel (available on FP10)
IMI Glucagon (available on FP10)
In doctor's bag
Hypostop gel
IMI Glucagon.
IV Dextrose.

Materials/resources for diabetes education

Items 1-5 are often available from pharmaceutical companies (see resources list Chapter 16 for addresses).

1. **Posters** – Give information. Useful as educational aids on specific topics.

2. **Information booklets/leaflets** – for individual and appropriate use.

3. **Videos** – for education sessions.

4. **Self monitoring diaries.**

5. **Identification cards.**

6. **Local diabetes units/centres** – contact numbers.

7. **British Diabetic Association** – national organisation. Local branches for adults and parent groups – contact numbers.

8. **Local information and contact numbers for:**
   - i   Chiropody services
   - ii Dietetic services
   - iii Dental services
   - iv Pharmacy services
   - v   Optician services
   - vi Supporting/caring agencies/trusts
   - vii Social services and benefits
   - viii Rehabilitation services

9. **Further information** – may be required for:
   Shopping (eg specific foods, shoe fitting)
   Leisure facilities
   Travel/holidays (eg immunisation).

Materials for organisation and recording information

1. Diabetes register   } Perhaps held
2. Recall sheet/card index   } on computer
3. Appointment cards – for patient use.
4. Appointment book – to record appointments made.
5. Standard letter – for use for new patients attending.
6. Card/leaflet – with practice information and practice contact numbers.

7. Laboratory forms.

8. Patient's medical records.

9. Diabetes record of care (held by the person with diabetes or the practice; perhaps held on computer).

Recording information

Individual diabetes record of care (see Fig 4.1)

1. Every person with diabetes should have their care recorded. This should include at least:

    i demographic information.

    ii a record of clinical checks and results.

    iii a record of education topics covered.

    iv a record of treatment targets and management.

    v a record of particular problems and actions taken (or to be taken).

2. Where the information is to be recorded requires discussion and a practice decision. The options might be:-

    i Information recorded on computer – printed out – practice medical record (this will make the medical records bulky).

       Note It is necessary for a written record of care to be made for medico-legal purposes.

    ii Information recorded in practice medical records.

    iii Information recorded in Diabetes Record Card (practice held).

    iv Information recorded in Diabetes Record Card (patient held) *and* in practice medical records or in Diabetes Record Card (practice held).

3. Should any problem or question arise regarding the care of a patient, the diabetes record is the *only* demonstration of care provided (particularly if care is only provided by the practice).

4. Diabetes Record (co-operation) Cards may:

    i Be provided by the district.

    ii Provided by pharmaceutical companies (eg Boehringer Mannheim).

    iii Designed by individual practices for their own use.

Practice information relating to diabetes care provision

In order to assess the health needs of the practice population and for the short and long term planning of the practice diabetes service, the recording of information is necessary for the following reasons:

1. To monitor the diabetes service.

2. To evaluate diabetes care provided.

3. To obtain statistical information (eg epidemiological, medical – see Chapter 15).

Fig 4.1 Sample Diabetes Record Card designed by a practice team.

Diabetic Flow Sheet

SURNAME		FORENAMES	D of B	SEX

INITIAL ASSESSMENT	DIAGNOSIS
DATE:	
CVS	AGE AT
PULSES R L BRUIT	CRITERIA:
FEM.	
POP.	TREATMENT PLAN
POST. TIB.	
D. PEDIS	DIET
VISUAL ACUITY R L	WEIGHT
LENS	
FUNDI	DRUGS
WEIGHT	
STANDARD WT.	OTHER
HEIGHT	
CNS ⟨ VIBRATION / REFLEXES	FASTING B. S. ⟨
MSU	2 HR POST–P. B.S. ⟨
UREA/CREATININE	FAMILY & OBSTETRIC HISTORY
CXR	
ECG	
CHOLESTEROL	
Hb, FBC	TOBACCO ALCOHOL
TROPHIC CHANGES	

5 The symptoms of diabetes mellitus

The symptoms of diabetes are similar in both types of the condition. There are however certain differences between insulin dependent (IDDM) and non-insulin dependent diabetes (NIDDM). The two most important to remember are:

1. The rate of onset of symptoms
a) **Fast** in IDDM
b) **Slow** in NIDDM

2.a) Symptoms may be *present* but *unrecognised* in NIDDM by the patient or the physician.
b) Presenting symptoms in IDDM are more *obvious* to the patient but may not always be *recognised* by the physician.

Fig 5.1 shows the symptoms of diabetes as they occur in insulin dependent and non-insulin dependent diabetes and the similarities and differences between the two types of the condition.

Fig 5.1 The symptoms of diabetes mellitus.

SYMPTOMS	IDDM	NIDDM
Onset	Fast (Weeks)	Slow (Months, Years)
Thirst	✔	✔
Polyuria/nocturia	✔	✔
Incontinence in elderly	—	✔
Bed wetting in children	✔	—
Tiredness/lethargy	✔	✔

Fig 5.1 continued

SYMPTOMS	IDDM	NIDDM
Mood changes (irritability)	✔	✔
Weight loss	✔++	✔
Visual disturbances	✔	✔
Thrush infections (genital)	✔	✔
Recurrent infections (boils/ulcers)	✔	✔
Hunger	✔	✔
Tingling/pain/numbness (in feet, legs, hands)	___	✔
Occasionally, abdominal pain	✔	___
Unexplained symptoms	✔	✔

The signs of diabetes (ie those that can be measured) are shown in Fig 5.2. The presence or absence of glycosuria, ketonuria, fasting and random blood glucose levels for the diagnosis of diabetes can be seen.

Fig 5.2 Signs of diabetes mellitus (that can be measured).

SIGNS	IDDM	NIDDM
Glycosuria	Present	May be absent
Fasting blood glucose	Venous or capillarywhole blood **greater than 8 mmol/l**	
Random blood glucose	Venous or capillary whole blood **greater than 11 mmol/l**	
Ketonuria	May be present	Usually absent

Public awareness of diabetes

Symptoms and signs of insulin dependent diabetes are usually acute and the diagnosis should be made quickly, once the patient or family seek advice.

Many people with non-insulin dependent diabetes live with the condition undiagnosed for months or years before seeking advice, by which time complications are well established.

The general public may well know 'something' about diabetes. This is often that diabetes is associated with 'sugar'. The nature of the association, however, is not necessarily understood. More important, the symptoms are not known, or because of their non-specific nature, are not related to the diagnosis of diabetes.

Symptoms of tiredness or lethargy may be explained away by 'I'm getting older'; irritability, by stress at work or in the home. Repeated infections may be treated by different doctors in a large practice and the significance of their frequency not realised. Symptoms may also occur or progress so slowly and in such a 'mild' way that they are not connected to NIDDM.

Improving public awareness of diabetes

1. All members of the public are registered with a doctor (or should be). The primary care team in the practice should always have 'diabetes' in their thoughts when providing any health care.

2. Posters (see Fig 5.3) can be put up in surgeries and waiting areas showing the symptoms of diabetes:

Fig 5.3 Poster showing symptoms of diabetes – for surgery use.

DIABETES – DO YOU SUFFER FROM

- Excessive thirst?
- Going to the toilet to pass water (a lot)?
- Visual changes?
- Genital irritation?
- Lethargy?
- Weight loss?
- Mood changes?
- Weight gain?

IF SO PLEASE LET US KNOW

3. Health questionnaires used in routine screening or for new patients to the practice should contain questions about symptoms of diabetes (as shown in the sample poster, Fig 5.3).

Screening for diabetes mellitus

Mass screening for the detection of diabetes entails considerable organisation and costs. However, screening of certain groups of people at risk is feasible and cost effective. An opportunistic, routine or 'on suspicion' approach should be adopted.

The following figure (Fig 5.4) shows who should be screened, who could be screened and the opportunities available for screening.

Fig 5.4 Candidates for screening.

Opportunities for screening	Should be screened	Could be screened
By the primary care team	Symptoms	People more likely to develop diabetes
During surgery	Thirst	
In health promotion clinics	Polyuria/nocturia	Family history (of diabetes mellitus)
New patients to the practice	Bed wetting in children	Overweight
In 'home' screening programmes (eg the elderly)	Incontinence in elderly	Elderly
	Weight loss (Sudden or gradual)	Asian/Afro-Caribbean
At routine medical checks (eg insurance)	Lethargy	Pregnant
	Mood changes	Previous gestational diabetes
	Persistent infections (boils, abscesses, slow healing ulcers)	Obstetric history (babies >4 kg, unexplained foetal loss)
	Visual changes	Presence of peripheral vascular disease
	Symptoms of neuropathy/ pins and needles in feet and legs	Cardiac problems
	Unexplained symptoms	Circulatory problems

Diagnosis of diabetes mellitus

Important notes

1. Confirmation of urine test - positive for glucose
Should a urine test reveal the presence of glucose, it is important that further tests are carried out for fasting and/or random blood glucose levels (or by oral glucose tolerance test), as glycosuria may be due to a LOW renal threshold.

Consequently, the diagnosis of diabetes may be missed in an older person with a HIGH renal threshold (the urine test may show a NEGATIVE result, where the blood glucose level is 13 mmol/l or more).

2. The Renal Threshold
The renal threshold (see Fig 5.5) is the level at which glucose spills over into the urine as blood glucose levels rise. A normal renal threshold is approximately 10 mmol/l (ie when the blood glucose level is measured it is 10 mmol/l and glycosuria is detectable). The renal threshold usually rises with age so that high blood glucose levels are present in the absence of glycosuria. The renal threshold may be low in some people and particularly during pregnancy (see Fig 5.5).

3. Telling the patient
Once glycosuria has been found, the patient should be told of this and that further tests are required for the following reasons:

a) The patient may *not* have diabetes but may have a low renal threshold (eg in pregnancy).
b) The patient has diabetes (if pregnancy - gestational diabetes).
c) The patient has impaired glucose tolerance.

Reassurance of the patient is important and confirmation of the diagnosis should be made as quickly as possible in order that appropriate treatment, support and education can begin. Preconceived ideas, fear and anxiety surround a diagnosis of diabetes. Firm evidence and careful explanation are essential, whether a diagnosis is confirmed or not.

Confirming the diagnosis

A diagnosis of diabetes may be confirmed by a random laboratory venous blood glucose values ≥ 11 mmol/l and/or a fasting laboratory venous blood glucose value ≥ 8 mmol/l. Where the diagnosis is in doubt (or there may be impaired glucose tolerance) an oral glucose tolerance test (OGTT) should be performed.

Fig 5.5 The renal threshold.

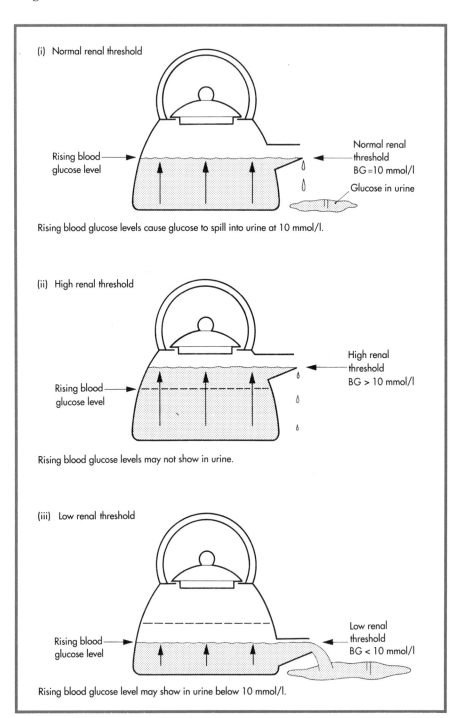

(i) Normal renal threshold

Rising blood glucose level

Normal renal threshold
BG = 10 mmol/l

Glucose in urine

Rising blood glucose levels cause glucose to spill into urine at 10 mmol/l.

(ii) High renal threshold

Rising blood glucose level

High renal threshold
BG > 10 mmol/l

Rising blood glucose levels may not show in urine.

(iii) Low renal threshold

Rising blood glucose level

Low renal threshold
BG < 10 mmol/l

Rising blood glucose level may show in urine below 10 mmol/l.

The hearty breakfast test

If the patient attends the surgery following an overnight fast, a laboratory venous sample (for blood glucose) can be obtained. Following this, a 'hearty breakfast' (see Fig 5.6) is eaten (at home by the patient!) followed by a second laboratory venous blood sample (for blood glucose) taken 2 hours later.

Fig 5.6 A hearty breakfast menu.

- **Fruit juice**
- **Cereal and milk (with sugar if taken)**
- **Coffee or tea (with sugar if taken)**
- **Cooked breakfast (eggs, bacon etc, if liked)**
- **Toast and marmalade**

Note An alternative to the 'hearty breakfast' would be 375 ml of Lucozade (supplied by the patient) and a venous blood sample taken 2 hours later.

Impaired glucose tolerance

Impaired glucose tolerance (IGT) is indicated by a fasting laboratory venous blood glucose value ≥ 7 mmol/l and ≤ 10 mmol/l. Confirmation of IGT is made by the performance of an oral glucose tolerance test (OGTT).

Oral glucose tolerance test (OGTT)

WHO recommendation

The OGTT is used principally for diagnosis when blood glucose levels are doubtful, during pregnancy, or to screen for diabetes and impaired glucose tolerance in an epidemiological setting.

The test

1. The test should be administered in the morning, following at least three days of unrestricted diet (greater than 150 g of carbohydrate daily, ie full daily meals and snacks including bread and potatoes) and usual physical activities.

2. The test should be preceded by an overnight fast (10-16 hours) during which water may be drunk.

3. Smoking is not permitted during the test.

4. Factors influencing interpretation of the test should be recorded (eg infection, inactivity, medications).

5. A fasting venous blood sample should be collected first. 'Fasting' and the time should be noted on the accompanying form.

6. The patient is then given 75 g of glucose in 250-300 ml of water (PLJ – lemon juice – may make this more palatable, as patients often find the glucose solution nauseating). Alternatively 375 ml Lucozade may be used. The glucose solution or Lucozade should be taken over approximately 5 minutes. The drink is more palatable taken through a straw.

7. A venous blood sample should be taken 2 hours after the glucose load (samples may also be taken at half-hourly intervals during this period, for a more detailed profile).

8. The accompanying laboratory form(s) should state the time of the glucose load and the collection time of the blood sample.

9. Samples should be sent straight to the laboratory following completion of the test.

In summary

Confirming the diagnosis of diabetes mellitus

	No diabetes	Diabetes	Impaired glucose tolerance
Fasting blood glucose	≤ 6	≥ 8	≤ 7
Random blood glucose (2 hours after glucose load)	≤ 8	≥ 11	≥ 7 ≤ 10

Note Capillary whole blood glucose values are 1-2 mmol higher than venous whole blood glucose values.

Identification of people with diabetes

Details of people newly diagnosed with diabetes should be noted on a register (computer or written), as should those identified with diabetes and new to the practice. People attending the practice who are already diagnosed with diabetes can be identified through records, prescriptions and at surgery attendance. Medical notes should be flagged following identification as (Diab).

Those treated with diet alone or who are housebound are more difficult to identify as they may not collect prescriptions or require, or be able, to attend the surgery for health care services.

Compiling a list

1. Practice staff and the primary care team need to 'think diabetes'!

2. Administrative staff (clerks/receptionists) should be educated about diabetes so that they can recognise the names of test strips, drugs and insulin on prescriptions and identify people from their treatment and monitoring strips.

3. A 'named' person should be given responsibility for the list. This person can also remind others in the practice to note names of people with diabetes seen in surgery, health promotion clinics, casual callers, people collecting prescriptions and prior to home visits. (Verbal reminders or 'reminder' cards on each desk may be required.)

4. Check existing knowledge of people with diabetes with doctors, nurses, administration staff.

5. Check existing registers.

6. Check prescription lists.

7. Check existing 'labelled diabetes' patient records.

8. Check patients new to the practice.

9. Note those newly diagnosed (from hospital, surgery, or home screening visits).

10. Be extra vigilant for people treated with diet alone.

11. Check records of regular home visits (for housebound).

12. Posters in surgery (see Fig 5.7).

Fig 5.7 Identification poster for surgery use.

Do you have diabetes?
are you treated with:

- **diet?**
- **tablets?**
- **insulin?**

For your care
please make sure
we know!
thank you

---

13. Maintain communication about diabetes with *all* members of the primary care team, especially those caring for the elderly and people suffering from mental illness/handicap.

14. Make contact with the local pharmacist(s) who may also have a list or knowledge of the local diabetes population.

15. Include any branch surgery population for total practice numbers identified.

To find out whether the practice has the expected prevalence (number of people with known diabetes), it is necessary to know:

1. The total population covered by the practice (total list size).
2. Percentage of elderly (ie those over 65 years of age) in the practice population.
3. Ethnic composition of the practice population.

A practice with a total list size of 2,200 people with a mainly Caucasian population and an average number aged 65 years or over would expect to have at least 1% (22 people) identified with diabetes. Approximately five of these might be insulin dependent and the remainder non-insulin dependent (treated with diet, diet and tablets, or diet and insulin).

Once identified, the name should be added to the list and the patient records labelled 'diabetes' (brown label, available from FHSA).

The list of names forms the basis of a 'diabetes' register (computer or written).

The practice diabetes register

It is required by the DOH that registers of people with diabetes are provided by every practice. District-wide registers are also developing. Requirements for these may be discussed and local guidelines should be followed. In order to provide a service for people with diabetes, a register is needed for the following reasons.

- To *know* how many people have diabetes in the practice.
- To *ensure* that care is available and provided for all people with diabetes in the practice.
- To *control* care provision, ie by the primary care team, hospital based team, if shared, or where care is inadequate.
- To *highlight* care provision that may be inadequate in treatment, education, support and surveillance. For example, where health care is provided by those with no special interest in diabetes, or where the person with diabetes may not be in permanent residence, eg students, businessmen, travellers, ethnic minority groups unaware of health care. People with diabetes treated with diet alone may also receive inadequate care.
- To *achieve the aim of organised individualised care* by knowing:
  a) The population with diabetes
  b) Where care is provided (and by whom)
  c) What care is provided
  d) The standard of care provision.

The register is invaluable in the 'tracking' of people with diabetes who fail to attend or do not attend hospital or general practice for their care, or who may be 'lost' between the two.

Setting up the register

1. Collect the list of names of people identified with diabetes.
2. Take out records – form list of names (include those at branch surgeries).
3. Note the following:
a) Name (address if required)
b) Date of birth
c) Duration of diabetes (not always possible)

d) Treatment – diet, diet and tablets, or diet and insulin

e) Identified complications of diabetes (or important associated medical problems)

Retinopathy

Neuropathy (peripheral/autonomic)

Nephropathy

Cardiovascular disease

Peripheral vascular disease

(This information will be available from hospital letters following clinic appointments).

f) Where care is provided eg specialist diabetes physician, other hospital physician, general practitioner, both or none. (The information regarding specialist/other physicians is obtained by checking the letter heading and knowing who the specialist physicians are in the district).

Fig 5.8 shows an example of a diabetes register.

Maintaining a diabetes register

1. A named person in the practice should take responsibility for maintaining the register.

2. Any changes (additions, deletions, demographic, treatment, complications or care provision) should be noted as they occur.

3. Training is required for a new person taking on the responsibility of the register.

4. The system devised for the maintenance of the register should be as *simple* as possible.

5. The register will form the basis of the follow up and recall system for diabetes care in the practice.

Links with specialist services

Before setting up the practice diabetes service, it is important to know where appropriate referrals to specialist services will be made, what diabetes services are available and the best way of obtaining them.

Contact with the appropriate diabetes team should provide the following necessary information:

1. The name(s) of the local diabetes physician(s) (diabetologists).

2. Names of diabetes nurse specialists.

3. Details of hospital diabetes clinics (where and when clinics are held) including collaborative clinics eg for foot, renal and antenatal care.

4. Name(s) of paediatrician(s) with an interest in diabetes.

Fig 5.8 Sample diabetes register.

	Name	Date of Birth	On Diet	On Tablets	On Insulin	Any Problems/Complications	Consultant Initials Hospital	Where Seen	
								GP	Both
1									
2									
3									
4									
5									
6									
7									
8									
9									
10									

Diabetes Register

5. Diabetes nurse specialist caring for children (may be separate or part of the diabetes nurse team).

6. Details of diabetes clinics for children including collaborative clinics eg for teenagers, young people.

7. Details of any district diabetes services provided for the elderly.

8. Details of availability and access to diabetes centres

a) by people with diabetes

b) by the practice team.

9. Advice, information and materials that may be identified as needed by the practice before setting up the service.

10. Information regarding self help groups for people with diabetes, eg local branches of the British Diabetic Association – for adults and/or parents/children.

11. Contact for the national British Diabetic Association.

Links with dietetic services

Obtain information on the following:

1. What district information is available regarding dietetic advice?

2. Who provides dietetic advice in the district?

3. What dietetic advice is provided for people with diabetes seen in the general practice setting?

4. Where and when are dietetic sessions available for people with diabetes, referred by the general practitioner?

Links with chiropody services

Obtain information on the following:

1. What district information is available regarding feet and shoe care?
2. Who provides chiropody services in the district?
3. Where and when are chiropody services available local to the practice (or perhaps they may be organised in the practice, either already for the practice population, or can people with diabetes be added in to an existing practice chiropody service)?
4. Who and where are private chiropodists (state registered) providing a service local to the practice?

Fig 5.9 Advertising the practice diabetes service.

Diabetes care

A new service for people with diabetes

- **to provide treatment, information and regular checks (if not provided elsewhere)**

- **held in this surgery**

- **every wednesday morning starting – 10.30 am (other times will be arranged if required)**

- **takes about 20 minutes**

- **appointment times given**

- **please ask at reception for details**

Fig 5.10 Example of a standard letter

Practice Telephone No: 222333
The Medical Practice
Woolly End Road
Airedale Edge
SHEFFIELD
South Yorkshire

January 1994

Mrs P Johnson
The Tannery
Black Terrace
SHEFFIELD

Dear Mrs Johnson

We will shortly be starting a new service of health care for people with diabetes attending the practice. The service will include a review of treatment,
information and regular checks.

The service will be provided in the practice (address above) every
Wednesday morning, starting at 10.30 am (other times will be arranged if
required). The appointment should only take about 20 minutes.

We have made an appointment for you to attend on <u>Wednesday 14 April
1994 at 11 am</u>. Should this time not be convenient, perhaps you could let us
know (telephone number at top of letter) and we will arrange another time.

Please bring with you any written food plan (diet sheet) you have been following, your record of urine or blood tests (if you keep a record) and a fresh
urine sample.

We look forward to seeing you.

Yours sincerely

Dr A Smith   Mrs M Jones
General Practitioner   Practice Nurse

Links with other agencies

It may also be helpful to have available information on the following:

1. Local support groups (for many general health problems eg stroke support groups, Alcoholics Anonymous – addresses available from local or central libraries).
2. Prescription exemption; Disabled living allowance.
3. Opticians.
4. Shoe fitting services.
5. Health food shops (in case this advice is requested).
6. Dentists.
7. Care and after care services (for walking sticks, frames, commodes, continence supplies etc).

Advertising the practice diabetes service

Once the people with diabetes are identified and the service planned, notice of this needs to be given. This can be done a) by poster-targeting anyone attending the practice for health care (see Fig 5.9) or b) by letter to individuals inviting them to attend for diabetes care (see Fig 5.10).

6 Providing the service

Example guidelines for clinical management

Suggested protocol for initial assessment of newly diagnosed patients

Note 1 A patient who is ill, where ketonuria is present or blood glucose is greater than 25 mmol/l, requires hospital referral within 24 hours.

Note 2 Patients under 30 years of age, pregnant women and all those diagnosed with insulin dependent diabetes (IDDM) should be referred to diabetes centres/services for initial treatment and education.

Note 3 Children presenting with glycosuria should be referred to appropriate paediatric units.

Note 4 The protocol (items 1-17) should be carried out over several visits during a period of approximately 12 weeks. Baseline measurements for annual review will be available at the end of this time.

Note 5 Specific education and information about diabetes and self-management are not included in the following protocols (see Chapter 14).

Protocol

1. Enter patient details on practice diabetes register.

2. Discuss general aspects of diabetes, enquire about any family history and history of illness leading to diagnosis.

3. Listen and respond to preconceived ideas and anxieties. Establish existing knowledge of diabetes.

4. Discuss general health.

5. Weigh patient and measure height. Calculate body mass index (BMI) and agree target for ideal body weight.

$$BMI = \frac{\text{Weight in kilograms}}{(\text{Height in metres})^2}$$

6. Test urine for glucose, ketones and protein.

7. Measure blood pressure.

8. Test blood for glucose, renal function, HbA_1.

9. Consider measuring random or fasting cholesterol and triglyceride levels in people under 65 years. Ideally, these should be measured after a period of treatment since initial high triglycerides will fall to normal levels when blood glucose levels are better controlled.

10. Practices should carry out the following tests on diagnosis and annually if necessary:

- Full blood count
- ECG
- Liver function tests
- Blood glucose
- ESR or plasma viscosity
- Thyroid function tests

11. Give simple explanation of diabetes, and discuss any fears that the patient may have.

12. Discuss lifestyle in relation to diabetes; record drinking and smoking, advise strongly against the latter.

13. Examine for complications of diabetes:

- Lower limbs
- Peripheral pulses and sensation
- Visual acuity
- Fundoscopy with dilated pupils
- MSU – if appropriate

14. Discuss food, meal planning and initiate advice regarding eating plan (see Fig 6.1 and Fig 6.2).

15. Record information in the practice records and in diabetes co-operation cards, if used.

16. Arrange prescription (if required) and next appointment – regular and early reviews will be necessary until the patient has a good understanding of diabetes and metabolic control is achieved.

17. Notify information to district diabetes register.

Fig 6.1 A scheme for diagnosis and management of people with non-insulin dependent diabetes – the overweight (BMI >27).

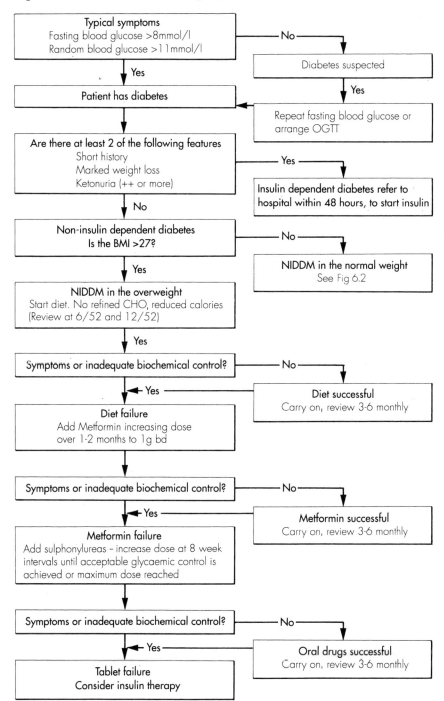

Fig 6.2 A scheme for managing non-insulin dependent diabetes – the normal weight.

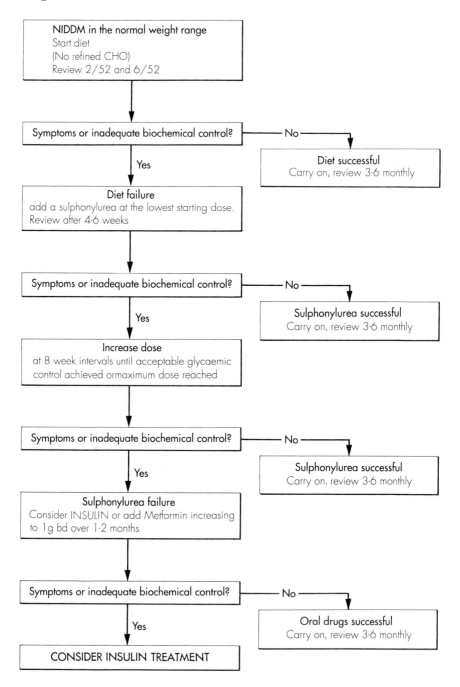

Example criteria for hospital referral

Referral is required in the following situations.

Urgent (telephone referral within 24 hours)

1. For protracted vomiting – an emergency referral is required.
2. Moderate or heavy ketonuria.
3. An acutely infected or ischaemic foot.
4. Newly diagnosed (insulin dependent)
5. Requiring insulin (non-insulin dependent)

Routine

1. If a pregnancy is planned.
2. If insulin treatment is required (referral should be URGENT in the newly diagnosed).
3. Problems in patient management eg if targets for control are not being met.
4. If complications are detected, eg;
   persistent proteinuria
   raised serum creatinine
   retinopathy
   unexplained loss of vision
   painful neuropathy, mononeuropathy, amyotrophy
   deteriorating condition of feet
   uncontrolled hypertension
   impotence

5. Psychological problems complicating diabetes, eg:
   failure to accept diagnosis
   morbid fear of complications
   family difficulties

Example protocol for performing a routine review

Ensure that patients with established diabetes are included on the diabetes register and are booked for regular appointments. A system for identifying and recalling defaulters should be organised and a policy agreed for the frequency of follow-up of people with diabetes. For routine visits where management and understanding of the condition are established and uncomplicated, these may only be required two or three times a year.

Protocol

1. Weigh patient (keep weight confidential, ie between patient and health care professional)
2. Test urine for glucose, ketones and protein; check MSU if protein present.
3. Take blood sample for HbA$_1$ (preferably take this sample (and any other blood samples) 7-10 days prior to review appointment so that results are available for discussion with patient).
4. Discuss the patient's general progress and well-being, enquire about any problems (life changes, diet etc). If treatment with insulin — check injection sites.
5. Identify and discuss any weak spots in knowledge of diabetes and self-management skills.
6. Perform examinations or investigations as required, (preferably 7-10 days before review appointment).
7. Discuss and agree targets with the patient – see guidelines below (Fig 6.3).
8. Record all details in diabetes record card and/or practice record.
9. Arrange next appointment.

Fig 6.3 A guide to glycaemic control – targets.

Biochemical indices of glycaemic control	Age (years)		
	30 - 50	50 - 70	Over 70
Fasting blood glucose under 8 mmol/l HbA$_1$ under 9%	Good	Depends upon their general medical health	Maybe over control/at high risk of hypoglycaemia on sulphonylureas/ insulin
Fasting blood glucose 8-11 mmol/l HbA$_1$ 9-10.5%	Undesirable but sometimes inevitable		Acceptable
Fasting blood glucose over 11 mmol/l HbA$_1$ over 11%	Undesirable	Undesirable	Undesirable but sometimes inevitable

Sample protocol for performing an annual review

Protocol

1. Weigh patient.
2. Urinalysis: glucose/albumin/ketones/microalbuminurea. Arrange MSU if protein/blood present.
3. Enquire about:

- subjective changes in eyes and feet
- claudication
- neuropathy symptoms, impotence
- chest pain, shortness of breath.

4. Examine for diabetic complications:

- blood pressure
- peripheral pulses and sensation
- lower limbs
- visual acuity
- fundoscopy with dilated pupils
- arrange MSU, if appropriate

5. Take blood sample for:

- blood glucose (feed back result)
- HbA$_1$ (performed in advance of annual review)
- creatinine
- cholesterol – this is recommended for those under 65 years of age, if found to be high at previous testing. (These tests should be performed in advance of the annual review.)

6. Discuss the patient's general progress and well-being, enquire about any problems relating to diabetes and whether any supplies are needed. If treatment with insulin — check injection sites.
7. Record information in the records and co-operation card if used.
8. Arrange prescription (if required) and next appointment.
9. Notify information to the district diabetes register.

Recall and follow up

People with diabetes (whether patients new to the practice or newly diagnosed), need to understand how the diabetes service is organised; the system of recall and follow up should be explained. Should an individual have a problem regarding attendance (due to employment shifts or family commitments), it is important that these problems are identified early on. The practice diabetes service should be sufficiently flexible to accommodate certain particular difficulties and incorporate visits for surveillance to the housebound receiving no other health care.

Where no system is in existence, the following procedure is recommended:

1. Note telephone number on records.
2. Use a standard letter (see Fig 5.10 in Chapter 5) inviting new patients to attend.
3. Agree a follow up appointment at the end of each visit.
4. Fill in an appointment card with the agreed date and time and give it to the patient before his/her departure.
5. Use a clinic diary (or card index system). Fill this in with the agreed times for each follow up visit to avoid over or under booking (a computer system may be useful here).
6. Allow enough time for each patient. Twenty minutes for a routine follow up visit, 30 minutes for an initial visit or an annual review.
7. Allow 5 minutes between each patient and 15 minutes (or more) at the end of each session for recording information and dealing with follow up work (such as organising dietitian, referral letters, chiropody).
8. Allow for a little leeway in each session if possible, for a person with diabetes requesting an unexpected or urgent visit.

Frequency of recall and follow up

Note It is not necessary for people with diabetes to attend the practice every week/month for the checking of blood glucose levels (except in unusual circumstances). A scheme such as this provides no benefit, it promotes diabetes as an illness and discourages self-management.

Frequency of recall and follow up may depend on the following:

1. Age, state and needs of the patient. These may relate to:

- being newly diagnosed
- being new to the practice
- discharged from hospital care
- requirement for help with losing weight
- feet at risk
- impaired vision
- mobility
- glycaemic control
- other medical problems (which may affect diabetes)

- education requirements
- support (emotional) (family/other problems)

2. Realistic recall targets relating to numbers to be seen in the practice cared for by practice team only and those receiving shared care.
3. Frequency of hospital appointments where care is shared.
4. Available transport.
5. Doctor/nurse time allocated/available.
6. Time of year relating to practice workload/annual leave by key members of team.

In a small practice, diabetes sessions may only be required monthly or even bi-monthly. A larger practice or a practice with a large number of people with diabetes (eg where there is a high ethnic composition), may require weekly sessions.

Specific sessions may be allocated for the annual review, or perhaps for visual acuity testing followed by fundoscopy where extra time may be required. Alternatively these may be carried out at the appropriate time in the year (at the same time each year) at a routine session.

The number of appointments for diabetes sessions or surgery visits *should not be excessive if sufficient time has been spent on clinical care and education.* Urgent or costly treatment may be avoided for the same reason.

- Every person with diabetes should be seen at least twice a year (every 6 months).
- People newly diagnosed or those experiencing problems may need weekly visits for a while, to incorporate baseline measurements and minimum education requirements.

Notes
- Elderly people with diabetes, sometimes with complications and/or multiple medical problems should be reviewed periodically in relation to visits to the practice, hospital or for other health care.
- It is important to ensure that time, cost and travel are not proving too great a burden and are truly beneficial to each person concerned.
- The recall and follow up system should be flexible and responsive to the needs of each patient, reflecting

Organised individualised care

Fig 6.4 An example of a practice annual recall system.

Sample
Practice Register, Recall And Follow Up
Year

Name	Date of birth	Jan	Feb	Mar	April	May	June	July	Aug	Sept	Oct	Nov	Dec	Foot check	Eye check	Home visit	New patient	New diagnosis	IDDM NIDDM both	H GP
																				H GP
1 Elsie Brown	10.2.20	C ✗		C FTA	✓									✓			✓		NI	GP
2																			NI	GP
3 John White	12.10.32		C✗ C✗ C✗	C ✓ ✓										✓	✓			✓	NI	GP
4																✓				
5 Freda Green	21.9.12				C✗		C✗ H				NB FIU✓			✓	✓	✓			NI	GP
6											✓									
7 Martin Black	15.6.80		C✗ H								✓			✓	✓			✓	–	H child
8																				
9																				
10																				

Key	✓ Due	C✓ Called	C✗ Seen	FTA Failed to attend

Reference

Heller, S R (1993) *Guidelines for clinical management.* Diabetes care in Sheffield FHSA Working Party/Diabetologists.

6

7 The treatment of non-insulin dependent diabetes mellitus

Aims of treatment

1. To relieve symptoms

2. To ensure a satisfactory lifestyle

3. To prevent unwanted effects of treatment (ie hypoglycaemia, side-effects of drugs)

4. To reduce the risks of acute complications (hypoglycaemia, hyperglycaemia)

5. To reduce the risks of long term complications

Relieving symptoms

Treatment should aim first of all to relieve symptoms. Assessment of symptoms should come before assessment of blood glucose control. Symptoms will decrease as blood glucose levels fall (these levels varying from person to person). People with diabetes soon learn the association between symptoms and hyperglycaemia and the benefits of treatment in renewed energy and an improved sense of well-being.

Ensuring a satisfactory lifestyle

People with diabetes and their families need sufficient information to make any lifestyle adjustments required by their treatment and monitoring, and to enable independence in their management of the condition. It is important that activity, exercise, eating habits, family and social life, and work are all considered in relation to suggested treatment.

Preventing unwanted effects of treatment (hypoglycaemia, side-effects of drugs)

Information should be given to the person with diabetes (relative or carer) regarding the effects of treatment, in particular the hypoglycaemic effects of oral hypoglycaemic agents. Information is required on the importance of:

- Regular eating
- Sufficient consumption of carbohydrate
- Monitoring of weight (by the person and/or the practice) as a reduction in weight may indicate that a lower drug dose is required.
- Noting and reporting symptoms of hypoglycaemia (see Chapter 10)
- Advice regarding prevention of hypoglycaemia (see Chapters 8 and 10).
- Side-effects of drugs prescribed (symptoms and that these should be reported to the care team).

7

Reducing the risks of acute complications (hypoglycaemia, hyperglycaemia)

Over treatment and under treatment should be avoided. Information should be provided regarding the following in relation to treatment prescribed:

Hypoglycaemia (for details see Chapters 8 and 10).
- Symptoms
- Treatment
- Prevention

Hyperglycaemia (for details see Chapter 10).
- Symptoms
- Treatment
- Prevention

Reducing the risks of long term complications

Risks to life and health in diabetes are due to
(a) recognised complications of diabetes,
(b) cardiovascular disease leading to premature death.

Minimising the risks of complications should include other factors as well as control of blood glucose levels. These factors are:

- No smoking
- Maintenance of a normal blood pressure
- Good blood glucose control
- Control of serum lipids

To achieve these the following are necessary:

- Regular medical examinations
- Support, education and advice in relation to treatment
- Individually negotiated targets for treatment and control
- Targets appropriate to age and ability to achieve them
- Regular assessment of symptoms and well-being.

In summary

1. Treatment must aim to alleviate symptoms and maintain the safety of the person concerned.

2. Simple risk factors should be reduced or eliminated.

3. Targets for control should be individualised and negotiated.

4. Sufficient information should be given to the person with diabetes (relative or carer) to understand their diabetes and achieve independence in its management.

Starting treatment (NIDDM)

Some important points

1. Assess preconceived ideas and knowledge about diabetes and treatment. Reassurance, support and information are needed. People with diabetes, newly diagnosed, are often concerned that they will be on a 'strict diet' for the rest of their lives or frightened that they will be 'on the needle'.
2. Explain that there are three types of treatment of diabetes:
  Modification of food intake (dietary habits).
  Modification of food intake and drugs.
  Modification of food intake and insulin.
3. Explain that treatment is ongoing and that it may be changed if symptoms persist and blood glucose levels remain high.

4. Emphasise that should a change in treatment beco[...] mean failure on the part of the person with diabetes.

5. Explain that the treatment is individually prescribe[...] and its effects are particular to each person.

Note 1 A young person, newly diagnosed with insulin [...] should be referred to the hospital based team.

Note 2 A guide to insulin therapy is provided in Chapter 8.

The treatment

- Treatment prescribed will depend on the age, weight, lifestyle and any other medical conditions of the person concerned (of particular importance in the elderly).

!WARNING!
- Patients should not be started on treatment with drugs before assessment of their weight, dietary habits and advice on modification of their food intake.

!WARNING!
- No treatment should be started before the diagnosis has been confirmed.

- Modification of food intake and dietary habits are the first lines of treatment in almost all cases.
- It is important, when planning treatment, to distinguish between people with diabetes who are of normal weight and those who are overweight.
- It is usually clinically obvious that the person concerned is overweight. However, a Body Mass Index (BMI) of greater than 27 indicates this condition – the formula for calculating the BMI is given in Chapter 6.

Note Examples of treatments schemes are shown in Fig 6.1 and Fig 6.2.

Dietary treatment

1. The 'cornerstones' of treatment are modification of food intake and dietary habits. These should be tried for at least three months before drug treatment is considered. Dietary advice, if followed, may well relieve the symptoms and improve metabolic control successfully.

2. Ideally, people with non-insulin dependent diabetes should see a dietitian for assessment and individual advice.

3. 'Stop-gap' advice, backed up with written information is acceptable initially.

4. The practice nurse or other designated members of the primary care team can give dietary advice, if appropriately trained.

…ss to a hospital based dietitian should be provided if no community …tian is available or if there is no trained member of the primary care team able to provide dietary advice.

Healthy eating and diabetes

- Modification of food intake is almost always the first line of treatment.
- The diet for a person with diabetes is not 'special', it is a healthy way of eating, recommended for everyone.
- It is important that an adequate and balanced nutritional intake is maintained (particular in an elderly person, who may have a diminished appetite).
- It is important to remember the social aspects of meal planning, shopping, cooking and meal time - in relation to family life. If there is a family life change (ie retirement, bereavement of a partner), this can have a profound effect on eating habits.
- 'Healthy eating' for diabetes is of benefit to all family members. Dietary advice should emphasise this point.
- No 'special' arrangements are required, adaptations to the usual food eaten are all that is needed.

Recommendations for healthy eating and diabetes are given in the list suggested below in Fig 7.1. This list could be used in the surgery as a basic guideline or stop-gap advice.

A simple guide (see Fig 7.2) to diet and diabetes for a newly diagnosed person provides advice in more detail until a comprehensive assessment and advice can be provided, either by a dietitian or trained practice nurse.

Fig 7.1 Healthy eating and diabetes.

1. Avoid being overweight

2. Eat regular meals

3. Eat more carbohydrate and high fibre foods
eg whole grain bread, potatoes, beans

7

4. Eat less sugar
eg sweetened soft drinks, cakes, sweets, chocolates

5. Cut down on fat

6. Watch salt intake

7. Control alcohol intake

8. Avoid special 'diabetic' products
eg sweets, biscuits, jams - usually sold in pharmacies

Fig 7.2 A simple guide to diet and diabetes.

1. Avoid sugar and sugary foods

- Do not add sugar to any food or drink
- Avoid all sweetened drinks, jams, marmalade and honey
- Avoid sugary sweets, biscuit, cakes, sweets, chocolates and 'diabetic' alternatives
- Instead, use low calorie and sugar free drinks. You may use sugar free artificial sweeteners (saccharin, Nutrasweet, Candarel, Sweetex plus)

2. Eat plenty of fibre

- Good sources are whole grain bread, whole grain breakfast cereals, fruit, vegetables, potatoes, brown rice and wholemeal pasta

3. Eat less fat

- Grill food rather than fry
- Eat lean meat and remove visible fat
- Cut down on butter, margarine, oil, lard and cheese

4. Eat regularly

- Do not miss meals
- Take a small snack between meals, such as a plain biscuit, a glass of semi-skimmed milk, a piece of fruit or a slice of bread or toast and low fat spread

(Produced by Sheffield Health Authority Dietitians 1990)

The British Diabetic Association dietary recommendations for people with diabetes

These can be summarised as follows.

Calories
- Keep calorie intake fairly constant (weight variation is an indicator of this).
- Fluctuations of calorie intake may have an effect on blood glucose levels.
- Eat regularly.
- Foods high in calories, such as fatty meat, fried foods, dairy products and sugary-foods and drinks can cause deterioration in blood glucose control.

Carbohydrate
- At least half of the calorie intake should come from carbohydrate foods such as bread, potatoes, rice, pasta, cereals, beans and lentils.
- High fibre varieties (such as whole grain bread, jacket potatoes) should be used.
- Beans, lentils, oats and citrus fruits have been shown to promote a slow, steadier rise in blood sugar levels.
- Rapidly absorbed carbohydrate foods (eg sweets, chocolates, sweet drinks) should be kept for special occasions, emergencies such as hypoglycaemia or illness, or as a snack before strenuous activity.
- Special advice may be necessary should a carbohydrate allowance be required. Changes should be kept to a minimum and advice obtained before they are made (eg when weight reduction is required).

Fat
- Eat less fatty red meat and meat products; eat more fish and poultry.
- Eat fewer dairy products eg cheese, butter, cream.
- Use a low fat spread instead of butter or margarine.
- Use skimmed or semi-skimmed milk instead of whole milk. Skimmed milk has fewer calories but some people find that semi-skimmed milk tastes better.

Salt
Reduce salt intake by:
- Eating fewer salty foods, such as pre-cooked meats, smoked fish or cheese.
- Add less salt during cooking.
- Cut down on salt added at the table.

Alcohol
- A maximum of three standard drinks for men and two standard drinks for women per day is recommended, following consultation with a physician.
- It is better to drink less alcohol. If weight is a problem, consumption should be limited to one drink per day.

- Calories should be counted into the overall intake
- 1 standard drink = half pint of ordinary beer or lager = a single measure of spirits (whisky, gin, bacardi, vodka, etc) = a glass of wine = a measure of vermouth or aperitif.
- Low carbohydrate beers and lagers should be avoided. These are high in calories and in alcohol.
- Alcohol lowers the blood sugar, so it is important not to drink on an empty stomach. Meals or snacks should not be replaced with alcohol.

Special diabetic foods
- These are *not* recommended. They contain no less fat or calories than other foods and may be low in fibre.
- Sorbitol is used to sweeten them and this may cause diarrhoea.
- Fructose may also be used in diabetic products. This has the same energy value as sugar. No more than 25 g/day should be taken.
- A small piece of ordinary (sweetened) cake or chocolate on the odd occasion, preferably taken at the end of a high fibre meal, is not likely to be harmful. Again, calories and carbohydrates should be counted in.
- Foods lower in energy content than their sweetened equivalents, such as low calorie squashes, diet fizzy drinks, diet yoghurts, fruit tinned in natural juice and artificial sweeteners should be used.
- Diabetic squashes are no better than low calorie squashes found in most supermarkets.

Important
- *Diabetic foods are expensive and unnecessary*
- British Diabetic Association recommendations regarding the use of sugar – if the person with diabetes is not overweight and follows a high starchy carbohydrate, high fibre, low fat diet up to 25 g of sugar can be used a day. This should be spread throughout the day and should not be used in drinks or on cereals where artificial sweeteners can be used.

Note
Further helpful hints, recipes and cooking tips are available from local dietitians and the British Diabetic Association, including special cultural modifications eg for the Asian or Afro-Caribbean person with diabetes.

Schedule of dietary treatment for people with non-insulin dependent diabetes who are overweight
- Assess food and alcohol intake (types of food and alcohol enjoyed and amounts taken during the day).
- Assess activity/exercise taken (on a daily basis).

- Discuss targets for weight loss - short and long term. These targets should be realistic, possible and desired by the person with diabetes.
- Provide appropriate advice.
- Monitor and support regularly, eg monthly if weight loss is not seen within three months and blood sugar remains elevated.

Schedule of dietary treatment for people with non-insulin dependent diabetes who are of normal weight
- Assess food and alcohol intake (types of foods and alcohol enjoyed and amounts taken during the day).
- Assess activity/exercise taken on (a daily basis).
- Discuss targets for maintaining weight - short and long term.
- Provide appropriate advice.
- Encourage regular activity and exercise.
- Monitor at regular intervals to check on weight regulation and blood sugar control.

Activity for health
- An active life and daily exercise are important in maintaining health and in the regulation of blood glucose control.
- Advice about exercise should be realistic and possible and should include information on local facilities available (eg swimming, health clubs).
- Information provided should include costs, which may be prohibitive for some people.
- Advice regarding exercise (particularly for those unused to it), should only be given in association with a medical examination and advice.

References

British Diabetic Association Report (1992). *Dietary Recommendations for people with diabetes.* Diabetic Medicine 9:189-202.

Department of Nutrition and Diabetes (1990). *Community Nutrition Information.* Sheffield Health Authority.

The Research Unit, Royal College of Physicians, British Diabetic Association and Royal College of General Practitioners (1993). *Guidelines for good practice in the diagnosis and treatment of non-insulin dependent diabetes mellitus.*

8 Drug and insulin therapy

Oral medication

Healthy eating through modification of food intake may be sufficient to achieve the aims of treatment in non-insulin dependent diabetes.

If symptoms persist and blood glucose levels remain elevated, oral medication may be required in addition to the dietary recommendations suggested.

Information regarding oral medication should include the following:

- The name of the drug
- The dose to be taken
- When to take the drug (ie before or at meal times)
- Hypoglycaemic effect of drug (sulphonylureas)
- Side-effects of the drug
- Possible interactions with other drugs taken
- What to do if problems occur (ie contact doctor or practice nurse)
- How to obtain prescription exemption (DOH Form No P11, to be signed by a doctor).

Oral hypoglycaemic agents

There are two main groups of drugs used in the treatment of non-insulin dependent diabetes. They are:

- sulphonylureas
- biguanides

In addition there is guar gum (not commonly used).

Sulphonylureas
Action
- Stimulate release of insulin from the pancreas.
- Increase sensitivity of peripheral tissue to circulating insulin.

Note As insulin is anabolic, the use of sulphonylureas (see Fig 8.1) may be associated with weight gain.

Fig 8.1 Sulphonylureas most commonly used.

Drug	Tablet size	Dose
Chlorpropamide (Diabenese)	100 mg or 250 mg	100 mg - 500 mg (once daily only)
Glibenclamide (Daonil, Euglucon)	2.5 mg or 5 mg	2.5 mg – 15 mg (once daily or in divided doses)
Gliclazide (Diamicron)	80 mg	40 mg - 320 mg daily (80 mg as single daily dose; higher doses divided)
Glipizide (Glibenese)	5 mg	2.5 mg - 30 mg daily (10 mg as single dose; higher doses divided)
Gliquidone (Glurenorm)	30 mg	15 mg - 180 mg daily (up to 60 mg as single dose with breakfast; higher dose divided with meals)
Tolazamide (Tolanase)	100 mg or 250 mg	100 mg - 1 g daily
Tolbutamide (Rastinon)	500 mg	500 mg - 2 g daily (divided doses)

Sulphonylureas – usage
- Sulphonylureas should be used for people with NIDDM of *normal weight* who are unable to achieve control of blood glucose levels by diet modification.
- Glibenclamide (Daonil, Euglucon) is the most popular of the sulphonylureas. It can however cause *significant hypoglycaemia*, particularly in the *elderly* or those with *renal dysfunction.*

- Gliclazide (Diamicron) is perhaps the most commonly used. It is excreted in the bile and can therefore be used in renal insufficiency. It is less prone to cause hypoglycaemia in the elderly.
- Tolbutamide (Rastinon) is safe and effective (particularly in the elderly) - though the tablets are large and may be difficult to swallow.
- Chlorpropamide (Diabenese) is *outdated*. It has a long duration of action and a tendency to cause hypoglycaemia.
- Sulphonylureas are potent drugs - and can cause profound hypoglycaemia which may be fatal. This problem is most common with the use of Glibenclamide (particularly where it is used in the elderly or those with renal dysfunction).
- Glibenclamide should not be used in those over 70 years of age or where there is renal impairment. Gliclazide or Tolbutamide are safer alternatives.
- Should hypoglycaemia occur, the drug should be substantially reduced or withdrawn.

Sulphonylureas - cautions, contraindications
- Encourage weight gain
- Should *not* be used in pregnancy
- Should *not* be used during breast feeding
- Should be used with *caution in the elderly* (because of dangers of hypoglycaemia)
- Should *not* be used in those with renal impairment

Note Tolbutamide, Gliquidone and Gliclazide may be used in renal impairment as they are metabolised and inactivated in the liver.

Sulphonylureas - side-effects
- Usually mild and infrequent
- Gastro-intestinal disturbances
- Headache
- Facial flushing following alcohol consumption (mainly Chlorpropamide)
- Sensitivity reactions (rashes)
- Blood disorders (rare) eg thrombocytopenia, agranulocytosis and aplastic anaemia

Biguanides
Action
- Unclear, but appear to decrease formation of glucose (gluconeogenesis)
- Increases peripheral utilisation of glucose.

Note 1 Metformin does not cause hypoglycaemia (except in large overdoses).

Note 2 Metformin to some extent *aids* weight loss.

Biguanides in use (in UK)

Drug	Tablet size	Dose
Metformin (Glucophage)	500 mg or 850 mg	500 mg - 3 g daily (divided doses with or after meals)

Metformin – usage
- Metformin should be considered in the *overweight* person with NIDDM who is unable to achieve control of blood glucose levels by diet modification.
- Metformin should be taken with food to minimise side-effects.
- Side-effects are less troublesome if small doses are used initially.
- Patients rarely feel better when treated with Metformin. Their well-being often improves following withdrawal of the drug.
- Risks of lactic acidosis have been exaggerated. These risks are considerably reduced if Metformin is avoided in the presence of hepatic, renal, chest or cardiac disease.

Metformin - cautions, contraindications
- Lactic acidosis (potentially fatal). However, this almost always only occurs where Metformin is used in people with renal failure.
- Metformin should NOT be used in:
    Renal failure
    Hepatic failure
    Heart failure
    Alcoholism
    Pregnancy
    Breast feeding

Metformin - side-effects
- Anorexia
- Epigastric discomfort/pain
- Nausea
- Vomiting
- Diarrhoea
- Lactic acidosis (IMMEDIATE WITHDRAWAL OF DRUG)
- Decreased Vitamin B_{12} absorption
- Unpleasant metallic taste

Guar gum (not commonly used)
Action
- If taken in sufficient quantities - some reduction in postprandial (following food) blood glucose levels probably by delaying carbohydrate absorption.

Note Guar gum is unpleasant to take.

Guar gum – usage
- Glucotard   ⎫ not
- Guarem   ⎬ commonly
- Guarina   ⎭ used

Guar gum - cautions, contraindications
- Gastro-intestinal obstruction.

Guar gum - side effects
- Flatulence
- Abdominal distension
- Intestinal obstruction

Combination therapy (sulphonylureas and metformin)
- Combination therapy (of sulphonylureas and Metformin) could be used where the person with NIDDM has been unable to achieve control of blood glucose levels on maximum doses of sulphonylureas or Metformin.
- This decision may be difficult and, in the interests of the person concerned, referral to a hospital diabetologist may be appropriate.
- The overweight person may 'improve control' when sulphonylureas are added to existing Metformin therapy - at the expense of further weight gain.
- The person of normal weight who is hyperglycaemic on the maximum dose of a sulphonylurea may have Metformin added to no good purpose, thereby delaying the use of insulin therapy which is urgently needed.

Insulin therapy

Approximately 25%-30% of people with NIDDM subsequently require insulin therapy for the following reasons:

- Insulin is obviously needed (where symptoms persist and blood glucose levels are high).
- Continuing weight loss (which may be gradual).
- Persistent ketonuria.
- In the presence of intercurrent illness.

Fig 8.2 Oral hypoglycaemic drugs – interactions with other drugs.

Drug affected	Drug interacting	Effect
Oral hypoglycaemic drugs	Alcohol, beta-blockers, monoamine oxidase inhibitors, Clofibrate, Bezafibrate, Gemfibrozil, Fenofibrate	Hypoglycaemic effect increased
	Corticosteroids, Bumetanide, Frusemide, Thiazides and oral contraceptives	Hyperglycaemic effect increased (antagonistic)
	Lithium	May impair glucose tolerance
Sulphonylureas (Chlorpropamide, Tolbutamide)	Chloramphenicol, Co-Trimoxazole, Miconazole	Hypoglycaemic effect increased
Chlorpropamide	Alcohol	Flushing in some patients
Chlorpropamide, Gliquidone, Tolbutamide	Rifamipicin	Reduced effect
Metformin	Alcohol	Increased risk of lactic acidosis
	Cimetidine	Increased plasma concentration of Metformin

Where insulin is obviously needed, where symptoms persist, blood glucose levels are high, weight loss has continued and ketonuria persists, the decision is clear. The introduction of insulin therapy will almost always relieve symptoms, lower blood glucose levels and improve well-being.

Where intercurrent illness occurs, insulin will be required for the following reasons (and others):

- Infections
- Increased insulin resistance
- Deteriorating blood glucose control
- Steroid therapy (increasing doses)

Note Following recovery, insulin is usually withdrawn and normal treatment re-commenced.

Trial of insulin

1. A three month trial of insulin may improve well-being and blood glucose levels in some people:

- where weight is stable
- who are unable to achieve targets for blood glucose control appropriate for their age or for other reasons.

2. Following a three month trial of insulin the person concerned should choose whether to return to oral medication or remain on insulin therapy.
3. Where the person with diabetes is overweight and poor blood glucose control persists, a decision to commence insulin therapy is more difficult.
4. Further modification of the diet is necessary.
5. A trial of insulin may be indicated, although in poorly controlled, overweight people whose food intake is excessive, gross obesity may result.

Aims for therapy

In younger people with NIDDM
The aim of treatment should be to improve blood glucose levels to reduce the risks of long term complications.

In older people with NIDDM (especially the elderly)
The aim of treatment should be to improve health and well-being.

Starting insulin therapy for people with NIDDM

- The person concerned will require considerable support, education and careful management.
- Specialist help (the hospital team) is recommended.
- An individual programme is required for stabilisation and continuing education.
- Blood sugar monitoring is almost always required if insulin therapy is

commenced, replacing urine testing – if previously used (see Chapter 10).

- Assessment of the capability, lifestyle and wishes of the patient is important when starting insulin, so that the insulin regimen allows a desired and appropriate lifestyle.
- A long acting insulin once daily, intermediate acting insulin twice daily or pre-mixed insulin twice daily may be used for older people.
- Visual aids, insulin pens and 'automatic' injectors may be required – if so, the hospital team should be consulted.

Insulin sources

- Insulin is extracted from pork and beef pancreata and purified by crystallisation.
- Insulin can also be made biosynthetically by recombinant DNA technology using *Escherichia coli.*
- Insulin can also be produced semi-synthetically by modification of pork or beef insulin.
- Human insulin (**emp**) Insulin produced by **e**nzyme **m**odification of **p**orcine insulin (**emp**), sometimes known as semi-synthetic human insulin.
- Human insulin (**prb**) Insulin **pr**oduced **b**iosynthetically (**prb**) by recombinant DNA technology produced from pro-insulin by genetic modification.
- Human insulin (**crb**) Produced by **c**hemical combination of a and b chains obtained from **b**acteria (**crb**) genetically modified by **r**ecombinant DNA technology.
- Human insulin (**pyr**) Insulin produced from a **p**recursor obtained from a **y**east genetically modified by **r**ecombinant DNA technology (**pyr**).

About insulin

- Human insulins (**prb**), (**crb**) and (**pyr**) are also known as biosynthetic human insulins.
- Insulin plays a key role in the body's regulation of carbohydrate, fat and protein metabolism.
- Diabetes mellitus is due to a deficiency in insulin synthesis and secretion.
- Insulin is inactivated by gastro-intestinal enzymes and must therefore be given by injection.
- It is usually injected into the upper arms, thighs, buttocks or abdomen, (there may be increased absorption from a limb site following strenuous exercise).
- Insulin is usually administered subcutaneously using a syringe and needle.
- Portable injection devices (eg Novopen, BD pen, Penject) hold insulin in cartridge form. The dose can be 'clicked up' and shown on a dial. Disposable pen

injection devices such as the Penmix 30/70 hold a larger reservoir of insulin and can be thrown away when empty.

- Pen devices allow greater flexibility of lifestyle although more injections are required where a multiple dose regime is used.
- Insulin can be given by continuous subcutaneous infusion (an insulin pump).
- When treating diabetic ketoacidosis, insulin should be given by intramuscular or intravenous injection, as absorption from subcutaneous sites can be slow and erratic.
- Minor allergic reactions at injection sites during the first few weeks of treatment are uncommon, usually transient and require no treatment.
- Rotation of injection sites lessens the chances of lipohypertrophy/lipoatrophy.
- Certain sites may become 'favoured' as their continued use lessens the discomfort of the injection.
- Insulin doses are determined on an individual basis (approx. 0.5 units – 0.8 units/kg body weight).
- Initial doses are small and gradually increased to avoid hypoglycaemia.

Three main types of insulin preparation

1. Those of SHORT duration which have a relatively rapid onset of action, namely soluble forms of insulin eg Actrapid, Humulin S, Humulin Velosulin. These can be given intramuscularly (IM) or intravenously (IV).

2. Those with an INTERMEDIATE action eg isophane insulin, insulin zinc suspension.

3. Those whose action is slower in onset and lasts for LONG periods eg Human Ultratard.

Note The duration of action of different insulin preparations varies considerably from one person to another and should be individually assessed before any dose adjustments are made. The monthly *MIMS Index* (Haymarket Press) contains a chart giving the onset, peak activity and duration of action of insulins.

Insulin – side-effect – hypoglycaemia

- Hypoglycaemia may occur when the patient's type of insulin is changed, eg converting from beef to human insulin.
- Therefore conversion from beef to human insulin should be undertaken with specialist advice.
- It is usual to reduce the total dose by at least 10%, with careful monitoring for the first few days.

- Careful monitoring is also required when changing from porcine to human insulin.
- Loss of warning signs of hypoglycaemia is a serious problem in people with diabetes treated with human insulin (particularly for drivers).
- Tight control of diabetes appears to lower blood glucose concentrations needed to trigger hypoglycaemic symptoms.
- Beta-blockers can also blunt awareness of hypoglycaemia (and can delay recovery).
- Some patients have reported a loss of warning of hypoglycaemia following transfer to human insulin. Patients should be warned of this possibility and if they believe that human insulin is responsible for their loss of warning, they should be transferred back to their pork or beef insulin.
- It is important that the type of insulin used by patients is clearly recorded.

Guideline for teaching self administration of insulin

Ideally, the person with diabetes requiring insulin therapy should have access to the hospital team. Considerable time, support, education and out of hours telephone contact/home visiting will be required initially and in a staged continuing process until confidence is gained and blood glucose levels stabilised.

Training and experience in 'starting' people on insulin therapy is required. Should there be no specialist team available and insulin therapy is indicated in an older person with diabetes the following guideline is provided; further points on education required are provided in Chapters 13 and 14.

The following steps are required:

- Assessment of the person with diabetes
- Preparation and support required
- Understanding the equipment
- Drawing up insulin
- Giving the injection
- Care of equipment
- Prevention of hypoglycaemia
- Treatment of hypoglycaemia
- Contact telephone number
- Identification
- Anticipation of problems and questions
- Evaluating learning.

Assessment

Language	For communication
Literacy	Understanding written material

Culture
Home, work, social conditions } Lifestyle

Hearing
Sight
Other medical problems
Physical state
Mobility
Dexterity } Physical ability

Mental state
Intellect
Preconceived ideas
Fear factor } Mental and emotional state

Preparation and support required

It is important to take into account preconceived ideas and fear (particularly of the needle). Emphasise the benefits of insulin, improved well-being and that support is available.

The benefits of insulin

- Direct action
- No need to take tablets (for diabetes)
- Feel better
- Improved lifestyle
- Lower blood glucose levels
- Risks of complications reduced

A 'dummy' injection

Experience of a 'dummy' injection by the nurse/doctor as well as the person with diabetes can be useful. Many people remember or imagine the needle to be large and that it is inserted into a vein. It may be helpful for the person concerned to meet another patient who has successfully transferred to insulin treatment.

An optimistic, helpful and positive approach is essential

Understanding the equipment

Insulin (bottle or cartridges)

Syringes (pen devices/needles)

Cotton wool

Needle clipper (discuss container for syringe disposal ie bottle with screw cap)

Educational material (leaflets on drawing up and giving insulin)

Insulin bottle or cartridges

TEACH

• Name and type
• Action – peak – duration
• Dose
• Expiry date
• Storage (bottle in use – spare bottle in fridge; pen devices should not be kept in fridge)
• Spare bottles/cartridges in fridge
• Prescription (check exemption)

Syringes (pen devices/needles)

TEACH

• Take to pieces
• Show how they work
• Explain types of syringe/markings (50 u-0.5 ml/100 u-1 ml)
• Demonstrate pen device/needle – correctly fitting together
• Air bubbles – how to expel
• Storage and re-use (one syringe/pen needle may be used for several doses).
• Prescription (required)

Cotton wool

TEACH

• Supplied by the person with diabetes
• Tissues may be used
• Used for gentle massage following injection

Needle clipper

TEACH

• Demonstrate
• Disposal (wrapped in household waste; syringes/pen needles in capped bottle in household waste or follow local arrangements for disposal)
• Replacement (obtained from GP or hospital clinic)
• Prescription (required)

Educational material
- Written leaflets
- Pictorial information

Drawing up insulin

TEACH
- The correct dose (write this down)
- How to draw up insulin correctly
- How to expel air bubbles
- When to give injection (20-30 mins pre-meal)
- Written leaflets (see resources list Chapter 16 and see Fig.8.3).

Fig.8.3 Examples of leaflets on drawing up, mixing and giving insulins – available from Becton Dickinson.

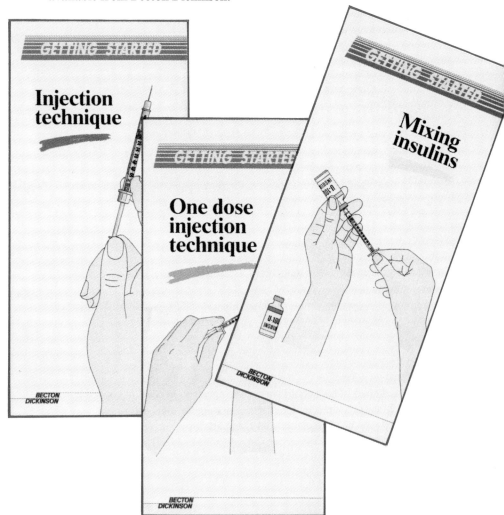

Giving the injection

TEACH

- Angle of injection (90° if normal/overweight; 45° if thin and skin pinched between thumb and fingers)
- Check dexterity (right or left handed; use of hands)
- Sites/rotation (insulin absorbed more quickly from abdominal site or in limbs following exercise). See Fig.8.4.
- Site for injection relaxed
- Massage gently with cotton wool/syringe following injection
- Encourage quick needle insertion (less uncomfortable)
- Encourage steady depression of plunger when injecting insulin
- Written and illustrated leaflets (see resources list Chapter 16)

Fig 8.4 Site rotation chart.

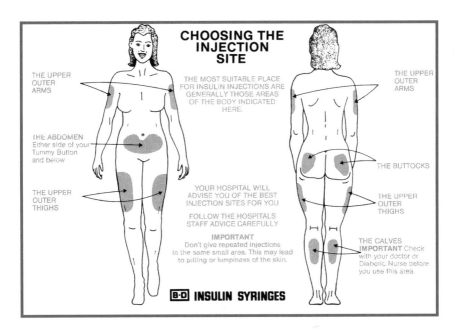

Care of equipment

TEACH

- Keep all together (with other equipment eg for monitoring)
- Always have a spare insulin (keep in fridge) bottle or cartridges
- Keep away from children
- List equipment required before attending surgery or hospital clinic – check insulin species, name, types of syringes used
- Re-use of syringes (pen device needles)
- Correct disposal (syringe/pen device needles)

Prevention of hypoglycaemia

TEACH

- Eat regularly (meals and snacks)
- Do not delay or miss meals
- Check dietary advice (refer to dietitian)
- Take correct dose of insulin
- Eat more carbohydrate (if activity increased)
- Less insulin needed (if strenuous activity anticipated)

Note Monitoring and education are required for self-adjustment of insulin.

- Carry glucose tablets/sweets – ALWAYS (keep in car – if driving)
- Inform DVLC – if a driver (new to insulin)
- Carry identification (necklace, bracelet or card) (see resources list Chapter 16)

Treatment of hypoglycaemia

TEACH

- Recognition of symptoms (pallor, sweating etc)
- Take 2-3 glucose tablets/sweet drink/sweets
- Follow up with substantial snack/meal
- Do not count this snack/meal in (it is extra to usual meals)
- Use of glucagon (by relative/friend – if unconscious)
- If driving – slow down, stop car safely – remove keys from ignition – move to passenger seat – treat as above
- Note possible reasons for hypoglycaemia:
  - ? too much insulin
  - ? insufficient food
  - ? delayed meal
  - ? more activity
  - ? stress
  - ? hot weather
  - ? new injection site used

Note There may (often) be no reason.

Contact telephone number

TEACH

- Surgery number
- Hospital diabetes centre/clinic number
- Out of hours number

Identification
TEACH
- Importance of personal ID
- Availability and source for necklace/bracelet (local jewellers or see resources list Chapter 16)
- Identification cards (BDA/insulin companies – see resources list Chapter 16)

Anticipation of problems and questions
EXAMPLES
Human insulin – does it come from humans?
- Reassure that this is not so. This may reflect concerns about AIDS (see section *About insulin* earlier in this chapter).

'Forgetting' the injection? What should I do?
- Advise – wait to give the next one, or two doses may be given close together (a hypoglycaemic reaction could result)

Giving the wrong dose? Too much or too little
- Explain action/peak/duration of insulin
- Explain effects of too much insulin – hypoglycaemia – recognition and treatment
- Explain effects of too little insulin – hyperglycaemia – correct at next dose, or seek medical advice if blood glucose levels high (a quick acting dose may be required)

Spirit for cleaning the skin?
- This is *not* required
- Makes injections uncomfortable
- Toughens injection sites

Bleeding following injection?
- Reassure this is nothing to worry about
- Check injection technique
- Apply gentle pressure to site if bleeding occurs

Evaluating learning
- At each stage following demonstration and teaching the person with diabetes/relative should demonstrate understanding
- Practical skills should be demonstrated
- Understanding evaluated by appropriate questions and in discussion
- Follow up appointments/home visits should be made at regular intervals until confidence is gained

- Monitoring is important once insulin therapy is commenced, in order to adjust insulin slowly to the appropriate level required for blood glucose levels, symptom relief and improved well-being
- Monitoring techniques require education and evaluation following the commencement of insulin therapy

References

The Research Unit, Royal College of Physicians, British Diabetic Association and Royal College of General Practitioners (1993). *Guidelines of good practice in the diagnosis and treatment of non-insulin dependent diabetes mellitus.*

Timmins, J G (1992). *Notes on Oral Hypoglycaemia Agents. Insulin Therapy.* Sheffield Health Authority.

9 Aspects of culture relating to diabetes care

Living with diabetes involves all aspects of life at any age and an understanding of culture is helpful in order to avoid giving inappropriate advice, causing misunderstandings or even giving offence.

- Religion and culture can vary greatly even within limited geographical areas.
- It is important to recognise family, social, local and country wide religions and cultural customs.
- Religious and cultural customs may change as people move from one stage of life to another (eg the child coming of age).
- Gender is of importance in many cultures.
- Hierarchy in a household may also be significant.
- Holy days or holidays involve a change in lifestyle for a period of time.
- Food is of great importance in all societies and the culture and customs surrounding it may be based on religious beliefs and should be respected accordingly.
- Religion may form the basis of the daily routine of prayers, work, relaxation and meal times.
- Certain foods (eg pork or beef) may be prohibited in some religions.
- Followers of religions may choose a devout and conservative path, while others may have a more relaxed view of the rules.
- Personal conscience dictates the choice of the individual as to which route they will follow.
- Cultural preconceptions should be avoided if possible.
- Understanding and respect for each individual is required.

Indo-Asian religion and culture

The prevalence of diabetes is particularly high in the Indo-Asian population in the United Kingdom, approximately four times higher than in the Caucasian population. Middle aged and elderly people tend to be more orthodox and conservative in their outlook than the younger generation. Extended families are common in the Indo-Asian culture. The mother-in-law may have considerable influence over cooking and shopping – important when dietary advice is given.

On moving to this country, many people of Indo-Asian origin change their environment and lifestyle, incorporating many 'western' features of food, meal habits and changes in activity levels (often taking less exercise than previously). Language may also prevent the women from moving out of the house, limiting their activity and access to health care and other benefits. Women may also be confined by their own culture and their role in child-bearing.

The younger generation have adapted quickly to a western culture, taking meals outside the home and consuming western food less nutritious than that traditionally eaten.

The Indo-Asian population consists of many religious and cultural beliefs. Cooking methods and meal times vary between groups and households.

The three main religious groups living in this country are:

- Hindus following Hinduism
- Moslems following Islam
- Sikhs following Sikhism

Hindus

Beliefs
- Life is a continuous process – all things are subject to reincarnation, birth, death and rebirth.
- A person is born into his caste – society is divided into different levels, linked to traditional occupations and to each person's duty in society.
- There are four main castes and within each caste, many sub-castes. Generally people marry within their own caste.
- Worship is mostly performed at home.

Festivals
There are two important festivals:
- *Holi* – February/March – 3 days
- *Diwali* – October/November

Food
- Many Hindus are vegetarian.
- Rich food is used at celebrations.
- Sweetmeats are consumed in large amounts.
- The cow is sacred to orthodox Hindus who do not eat beef.
- Women may fast for one to two days each week – this is not a total abstinence from food or drink. Some pure foods (fruit and milk) are allowed.

Moslems

Beliefs
- Moslems are the followers of Islam, which lays down social rules and religious behaviour.
- Moslems believe in Allah (one God) and that Mohammed was the last and greatest prophet.
- There are five main duties of Islam:
   i Belief in one God
   ii Prayer five times a day
   iii Giving $2^1/_2$% of annual income to charity.
   iv Fasting from sunrise to sunset during the month of Ramizan (Ramadan to non-Asians).
   v Pilgrimage to Mecca.
- Friday is the Moslem holy day.

Festivals
- *Ramizan* (Ramadan) occurs annually for one month. As the Islamic year is lunar (355 days) Ramadan falls 10 days earlier in the western calendar each year.
- *Eids* four or five times a year.
- Other festivals during the year.

Food
- It is against the Islamic religion to eat pork. Pork is regarded as unclean, and this should be remembered in the prescription of insulin; human insulin may be more acceptable.
- Orthodox Moslems may reject manufactured foods containing animal fat (lard).
- Many Moslems will only eat Halal meat (ritually slaughtered).
- During Ramadan, no food is taken between sunrise and sunset.
- A heavy meal is consumed before sunrise and again on breaking the fast.
- The old, the chronically ill and children under 12 years old can be exempt from fasting.
- Alcohol is strictly prohibited (as it results in loss of self-control).

Sikhs

Beliefs
- Sikhism is a reformist sect of Hinduism.
- Sikhs share many of their beliefs and ideas with Hindus.
- However, they believe in one God (not many, as do Hindus).
- The caste system is rejected.
- Devout Sikh families go to the temple (Gurudwaka) on a Sunday. The Gurudwaka is a focus for religious and community activity.
- Sikhs do not have family shrines at home.
- The five signs of Sikhism which unite and identify Sikhs are:
  - i *Kesh* – uncut hair including the beard (young men are clean shaven..
  - ii *Kangha* – a comb for men only to secure the hair under the turban.
  - iii *Kara* – a steel or gold bangle.
  - iv *Kirpan* – a small symbolic dagger.
  - v *Kaccha* – special undershirts worn by the men.

Festivals
- *Baisakhi* – Sikh New Year – this is celebrated by prayer and exchange of presents.
- The Birthday of Guru Nanak
- *Diwali* – celebrated by prayer and children receiving presents.

Food
- The temple (Gurudwaka) serves three free meals a day all year round.
- Most people eat one meal daily at the temple consisting of a vegetarian dish, chapatis and dessert.

Hot and cold foods

In many communities around the world it is believed that certain foods are 'hot' whilst others are 'cold'. The hot or cold nature of foods bear no relation to the temperature or to the spiciness of the dish. It is believed to be an inherent property of the food supposedly giving rise to physical effects in the body.

Hot foods are thought to raise the body temperature, excite the emotions and increase activity. Cold foods are thought to impart strength, cool the body and also to cause cheerfulness.

Normally a diet containing hot and cold foods would be consumed. However, during certain illnesses and in certain conditions, for example, pregnancy (which is a 'hot' condition) these beliefs assume a greater importance. During pregnancy, 'cold' foods would be consumed in preference to hot.

Some of the foods that are included in these two groups are listed in Fig 9.1.

Fig 9.1 Examples of 'hot' and 'cold' foods.

Food group	Hot	Cold
Cereal		Wheat Rice
Green leafy vegetables		All
Root vegetables	Carrot, onion	Potato
Other vegetables	Capsicum, pepper, aubergine or brinjal	Most other vegetables including cucumbers, beans, cauliflower, marrow, gourds, ladies fingers or okra
Fruit	Dates, mango, pawpaw or papaya	All other fruits eg apple, orange, melon etc.
Animal products	Meats – including chicken, mutton fish	
Dairy products	Eggs	
Milk products		Milk and cream, curds or yoghurt, buttermilk
Pulses	Lentil	Bengalgram or chickpea, greengram, peas, redgram
Nuts		All types including ground or peanuts, cashew nuts

9

Fig 9.1 continued

Food group	Hot	Cold
Spices and condiments	Chilli green and powder, cinnamon, clove, garlic, ginger, mustard, nutmeg, pepper	Coriander, cumin, cardomon fennel, tamarind
Oils	Mustard	Butter (ghee or clarified butter), coconut oil, groundnut oil
Miscellaneous	Tea, coffee, honey, jaggery or brown sugar	

Food modification and dietary advice

British Diabetic Association recommendations should accommodate the dietary culture and preferences for the Indo-Asian population. The general rules apply and should be individually tailored to the person, religion, culture and family circumstances. Specific advice and recipes can be obtained from the Chief Dietitian and Head of Diet Information Service, British Diabetic Association (see resources list Chapter 16).

Indo-Asian languages

The language of the person with diabetes must also be established along with the level of literacy so that information can be obtained in the appropriate language. Local ethnic groups and link-workers may also be helpful should translation be required.

Hindus speak Gujarati or Punjabi
Sikhs mostly speak Punjabi
Moslems may speak Gujarati or Punjabi
Pakistanis may speak Urdu or Punjabi
Bangladeshis speak Bengali

References

Brent Health Education (1986). *Religion and Culture: A Guide to Religious and Cultural Beliefs.*

Govindji, A (1991). *Dietary advice for the Asian diabetic.* Practical Diabetes 8;5:202,203

10 Control of blood glucose levels

Monitoring diabetes control by the primary care team

- The monitoring of the person with diabetes by the primary care team should support and check self-monitoring as well as ascertaining the effectiveness of treatment.
- Targets for control should be negotiated and realistic.
- Long term control can be confirmed by annual glycosylated haemoglobin or serum fructosamine tests.

Glycosylated haemoglobin (HbA₁)

The measurement of glycosylated haemoglobin is widely accepted as an objective and quantitative index of blood glucose levels during the preceding 6-10 weeks. This test is usually performed annually as an indicator of control over the period preceding the test. A fasting blood glucose level usually provides a similar result to the HbA₁ test. HbA₁ may be required more frequently where blood glucose control is poor. It should be remembered that the glycosylated haemoglobin test does not represent individual peaks and troughs in blood glucose levels. A low glycosylated haemoglobin or result within the normal range (4%-8% depending on the laboratory range) may indicate good control, though not reflecting levels of hypoglycaemia. Individual self-test results are also important and should always be discussed in any review of blood glucose control.

Serum fructosamine

An objective and quantitative test reflecting blood glucose control over the preceding 2-3 weeks only. This test is thus less useful as its time span is shorter. Fructosamine levels are used in some districts.

The benefits of monitoring

On diagnosis, following commencement or change of therapy and at any review, checks should be made on symptoms experienced (if any), ketonuria, glycosuria and blood glucose levels.

Confirmation of improvement in blood glucose levels, especially in the absence of symptoms (in NIDDM) will encourage continuity of self-care, treatment and monitoring.

Successful weight reduction will almost always improve blood glucose levels in NIDDM.

The success/failure of oral medication can be confirmed and medication adjusted if necessary.

A decision regarding the initiation of insulin therapy can be made.

Monitoring of dietary habits, changes in weight, lifestyle and other medical problems are also essential (particularly in the elderly) as any or all of these may affect diabetes control necessitating possible review and changes in treatment.

Monitoring by the practice team also involves urine testing for proteinuria, measurement of blood pressure and examination and surveillance for complications of diabetes, eg visual deterioration, retinopathy, foot problems (see guidelines for follow up and review Chapter 6).

High blood glucose levels (hyperglycaemia)

10

Hyperglycaemia is generally regarded to exist where blood glucose levels are above 13 mmol/l. This is certainly correct in a younger person with diabetes. For women who are pregnant, blood glucose levels should not rise above 7 mmol/l even following meals.

In older people however, especially where weight is a problem, blood glucose levels may be higher than 13 mmol/l. It is important that levels are discussed and that the person is symptom free.

Hyperglycaemia may be caused by:

- Untreated diabetes
- Too much food   } These may occur on
- The wrong type of food   special occasions!
- Insufficient medication (incorrect dose)
- Insufficient insulin (incorrect dose)
- Overuse of particular injection sites
- Poor injection technique
- Reduction of activity
- Decreased mobility
- Infections/illness

•. An increase in concurrent medication affecting glycaemic control (eg steroid therapy)
• Stress – life changes (retirement, bereavement)
• A weight increase.

Symptoms of hyperglycaemia need to be explained
Such as thirst, polyuria, nocturia (incontinence in the elderly), lethargy, irritability and visual changes.

Suggested changes and action to be taken
If the person with diabetes is self-monitoring it should be explained that occasional 'high' tests need not be acted upon. However, should hyperglycaemia persist, adjustments may be required (according to identified causes of the high blood sugar levels) regarding food/activity/medication/insulin. Particular action should be taken if an infection or illness disturbs blood glucose control.

Guideline for management of illness (by the primary care team)

• Monitoring equipment such as Ketostix and blood glucose test strips (in date and kept in airtight containers in a dry place, not in a fridge) and should be available in the surgery and in doctor's bag.
• Short acting insulin (eg Actrapid) may be useful to lower blood glucose levels in acute illness (in surgery and in doctors bag).

Guide for the physician
• Review therapy and treat intercurrent illness.
• Consider short term insulin therapy (for people usually treated with diet and oral hypoglycaemic agents).
• Refer to hospital if vomiting/hyperglycaemia/ketosis persists.
• Blood glucose control may deteriorate rapidly during an illness of any kind. People with diabetes require instructions on action to be taken during any intercurrent illness (see Fig 10.1).
• It is helpful if the relative or carer is also aware of these instructions in case the person with diabetes is unable to carry them out.
• The relative or carer should be able to draw up and give insulin if necessary and be able to monitor blood or urine glucose levels (if this is possible and appropriate).
• The person with diabetes/relative should have an emergency contact telephone number.

Fig 10.1 Illness rules: a guideline for the person with non-insulin dependent diabetes.

- A minor illness, such as a cold, may cause your blood sugar levels to rise.
- Blood sugar levels will return to normal once the infection is over, so usual treatment can then be resumed.
- Consult your doctor if the illness persists, if you have symptoms of high sugar levels or if you have high tests.
- Headaches and sore throats can safely be relieved using paracetamol or aspirin.
- Sugar-free cough remedies are available from your local pharmacist.
- Vomiting may result in you being unable to keep tablets down – Consult your doctor.
- Vomiting and diarrhoea may result in you losing a lot of fluid – Consult your doctor.
- You may need this fluid replaced.
- You may need insulin for a short time.

CONSULT YOUR DOCTOR

IMPORTANT RULES

- Continue with your diabetes treatment (diet and tablets or insulin).
- Ensure that you drink plenty of liquid (water, tea etc).
- Test urine or blood 2-4 hourly to check on how you are doing.
- If you are not hungry, substitute meals with a liquid or light diet (soup, ice cream, glucose drinks, milk – see Fig10.2 Emergency Exchange List)

- Consult your doctor in good time

10

Fig 10.2 Emergency exchange list.

If you are ill and unable to take normal food, the following amounts of food each contain 10g carbohydrate (one exchange).

Lucozade	2 fl ozs (50 ml)	—
Milk	7 fl ozs (200 ml)	1 cup
Fruit juice (natural unsweetened apple, orange, pineapple, grapefruit)	4 fl ozs (100 ml)	1 wine glass
Ribena – undiluted	1/2 fl oz	—
Ordinary squash	1 1/2 fl ozs	—
Coke or Pepsi	4 fl ozs (100 ml)	1 wine glass
Lemonade (fizzy)	7 fl ozs (200 ml)	1 cup
Glucose/sugar	—	2 level teaspoons
Complan	—	3 level tablespoons
Complan powder and milk	3 1/2 fl ozs milk	AND 1 1/2 level tablespoons Complan
Bournvita, Horlicks, Ovaltine, drinking chocolate	1/2 oz	2 heaped teaspoons
Porridge oats	4 ozs	4 tablespoons
Ice cream	2 flozs (50 ml)	1 scoop or small brickette

Fig 10.2 continued

Jelly (ordinary)	1/2 oz	2 tablespoons
Yoghurt (ordinary fruit)	2 1/2 ozs (75 g)	Half small carton
Yoghurt (plain)	5 ozs (150 g)	1 small carton

Note Thickened soups vary in content. 7 oz average serving contains 10 g carbo-hydrate.

Caution When measuring these concentrated carbohydrate foods make sure *standard* measuring spoons and *accurate* liquid measures are used. Gently level spoons with the back of a knife (do not pack into the spoons)

(Taken from Boehringer Mannheim's leaflet *When You're ill*)

Low blood glucose levels (hypoglycaemia)

- Hypoglycaemia is generally regarded to exist where blood glucose levels are below 4 mmol/l.
- It is important to remember that symptoms of hypoglycaemia may be experienced at levels higher than 4 mmol/l, in particular where blood glucose levels have been high for a period of time (eg following diagnosis).
- People with diabetes who strictly control their blood glucose levels are more at risk of hypoglycaemia.
- Hypoglycaemia can be delayed (many hours following extra activity).

Hypoglycaemia may be caused by:

1. Too little food } especially in
2. Delayed or missed meals } the elderly
3. Increased medication or insulin
4. Increased activity (exercise)
5. Increased mobility
6. A decrease in concurrent medication affecting glycaemic control
7. Stress – life changes
8. Hot weather (insulin treated – insulin absorbed more rapidly)
9. Change of injection site (where one site has been used repeatedly followed by use of a new site)
10. A decrease in weight (particularly in the elderly)
11. The prescence of renal failure

Symptoms of hypoglycaemia need to be explained
Such as sweating, pallor, headache, tingling of the lips, pounding heart, blurred vision, irritability, lack of concentration (confusion).

Diminished warning signs
Warning signs may not occur
1. In the presence of autonomic neuropathy, where diabetes has been diagnosed for many years (over 10 years).
2. Where strict blood glucose control exists.
3. Where repeated attacks of hypoglycaemia reduce significant symptoms.

The treatment of hypoglycaemia

Action to be taken
1. If the patient is conscious
- Give a sugary drink (use a straw) or glucose sweets (3-4) or sweets
- Give a substantial snack or meal (extra to normal meals)
- Check that blood glucose levels have returned to normal

2. If the patient is uncooperative
- Use Hypostop gel (available on prescription)
- Insert gel (approx. 1/3 of bottle) orally and massage gently around cheeks (the gel is absorbed into the buccal mucosa)
- Once co-operative – give a sugary drink or glucose tablets (3-4)
- Give a substantial snack or meal (extra to normal meals)
- Check that blood glucose levels have returned to normal

3. If the patient is unconscious
- Give glucagon injection (available on prescription)
- Place patient in recovery position and await return of consciousness (approximately 15-20 minutes)
- On recovery, sit patient up
- Give a sugary drink (use a straw) or glucose sweets (3-4) or sweets
- Give a substantial snack or meal (extra to normal meals)
- Check that blood glucose levels have returned to normal

Note 1
Should glucagon *not* render the patient conscious,

CALL THE DOCTOR

or

EMERGENCY SERVICES – DIAL 999

Note 2
Glucagon can cause vomiting.

Note 3
The patient may feel very cold on regaining consciousness.

Self monitoring in diabetes care

- When appropriate, following diagnosis and if they are able, people with diabetes should become accustomed to monitoring their own health.
- In a broad sense, this includes general health and well-being, diabetes control, eyesight, weight, dental care, care of the feet and footwear.
- In order to promote health and reduce risks of complications, the monitoring of diabetes control (urine/blood glucose levels) requires particular attention and involves careful assessment and education by the care team.
- Self-monitoring allows the person with diabetes to check their own control, take responsibility for their own condition and maintain independence (as far as possible).
- Four stages are required in the process of initiating a self-monitoring programme.

10

Stage I – Assessment
Physical
Vision, colour vision, co-ordination and manual dexterity should be checked. If there are problems with any of these a partner, carer or the primary care team will need to monitor control.

Educational
Capability for understanding and retention of knowledge. Literacy, for back up written material, language and culture.

Attitudinal
The desire to self-monitor and take responsibility for own control.

Lifestyle
Fitting self-monitoring in with home, work, social life.

User ability
Ability to understand and take action on test results.

Stage II – Teaching

Teaching involves the person with diabetes/relative/carer
a) Learning the skill.
b) Recording the information gained.
c) Understanding the information gained.
d) Acting on the information where appropriate.

- Following an assessment, teaching should be adapted according to the needs of the individual and their capabilities.
- Explanations should be clear and in language that is understood.
- It should be recognised that some people will require more in-depth information.
- Numbers and times of tests should be negotiated.

Stage III – Evaluation

- Record teaching and information given.
- Allow time for discussion of self-monitoring and to answer questions about recorded results.
- Check testing technique by asking the person with diabetes/relative/carer to demonstrate a test when attending the surgery for review.
- Check understanding of tests, interpretation of results and any action taken.

Stage IV – Reinforcement

- On subsequent visits, ensure that monitoring is discussed.
- At least annually, check testing technique, understanding of tests, interpretation of results and any action taken.
- Show interest in tests and results.
- Be encouraging and supportive at all times.
- Do not make judgements on people who fail to carry out tests, record them or bring their records for review.
- Re-negotiate and encourage ALWAYS.

Who is monitoring?

- The person with diabetes
- The relative
- The carer

Why monitor?

1. To indicate that diabetes is controlled using urine or blood tests in order that urine/blood glucose levels remain within limits appropriate to the person's age, duration of diabetes, lifestyle and wishes (with the knowledge of risks of short term and long term complications of diabetes).

2. To indicate deterioration of diabetes control, in order that an appropriate treatment review can take place.

3. To indicate improvement of diabetes control following a weight, dietary, medication or insulin change or adjustment.

- In order to appreciate the reasons for self-monitoring, the person with diabetes needs to understand the factors affecting the rise and fall of their urine/blood glucose levels, including the associated symptoms, possible reasons, changes to be made and actions to be taken.
- Targets for testing and control should be appropriate and individually negotiated.

Urine testing

- Other than in children (to avoid excessive finger pricks), urine testing is of little use in insulin dependent diabetes.

- Urine testing is most commonly used in people with non-insulin dependent diabetes (the elderly, or in certain types of employment, where blood testing may be impossible to carry out).

Fig 10.3 Urine testing instructions for testing for glycosuria using Diastix (Ames) and Diabur Test 5000 (Boehringer Mannheim).

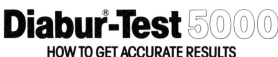

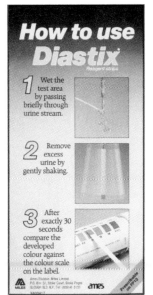

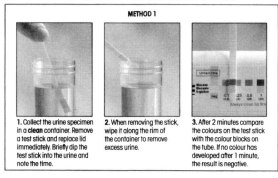

- Urine testing is inexpensive.
- The meaning of urine tests must be individually explained to each patient.
- A freshly passed urine specimen pre-breakfast, following early morning voiding, will indicate control during the day.
- Tests taken approximately 2 hours following a meal (2 hours post-evening meal) will indicate urinary glucose levels at their highest.
- If the renal threshold is individually explained, using a freshly voided specimen and a finger prick blood test (at the same time – in surgery) the person with diabetes will understand the meaning of their own urine tests and their relationship with blood glucose levels.
- A negative (or trace of glycosuria) urine test is the aim for older people, unless the renal threshold is found to be low.
- The renal threshold is usually equivalent to 10 mmol/l (blood glucose). This level rises with age.
- Often older people show negative urine tests but have blood glucose levels of 17 mmol/l or more (a high renal threshold).
- A negative urine test will not indicate hypoglycaemia, which may occur where older people are treated with sulphonylurea therapy.
- Should hypoglycaemia be suspected, (from discussion of symptoms or reports of 'dizzy do's'), blood sugar levels should be checked and medication or insulin reduced.
- Correctly *taught* and *timed* urine dipstick tests (see Fig 10.3) are simpler and safer than urine tests using tablets, which are caustic, messy and may be incorrectly used.
- A watch or clock with a second hand is required for home urine testing.
- Urine testing strips are available on prescription (free – except for people treated with diet alone, under the ages of 60 and 65 years of age – women and men respectively).
- The person with diabetes should be taught how to record tests and provided with a testing diary (available free – see resources list Chapter 16). These may also be obtained from the hospital clinic or centre.

Blood testing

- Blood testing is essential for people with insulin dependent diabetes, pre-pregnancy, during pregnancy or for those with gestational diabetes.
- Blood testing should usually be used by people with non-insulin dependent diabetes, treated with insulin.
- Blood testing may be used for people with non-insulin dependent diabetes, treated with diet or oral hypoglycaemic agents.
- Blood testing may be the monitoring method of choice by anyone with diabetes.

- Where people with diabetes are unable to self-monitor or use urine tests, blood testing is useful, even essential, to form a picture of day to day diabetes control. In these cases blood testing should be carried out by a carer or by a member of the primary care team. Such occasions might be:
    1. Where control is poor
    2. Where a treatment change is indicated
    3. To monitor a treatment change
    4. Where hypoglycaemia is suspected

Blood testing technique
- It is essential that hands are washed (by the person testing), preferably in warm water to encourage blood flow to the finger tips.
- Spirit swabs should not be used to clean the skin as the spirit may affect results.
- The side of the tips of fingers should be used (less painful).
- Fingers used should be changed at each test (to avoid discomfort).
- If the drop of blood is difficult to collect (into a 'tear' or 'tap' drop), Vaseline may be applied to the finger tip site prior to the test (this will accumulate the blood, stop it from spreading and will not affect the test).
- Finger pricking lancets can be re-capped and re-used.
- Lancets, following use, should be re-capped and dropped into a capped container (they may then be disposed of in household waste or according to local sharps disposal procedures).

10

Interpretation of results – action to take
- Blood tests taken pre-meal and pre-bed will indicate control.
- One blood test each day, taken at a different time will provide a blood glucose profile over several days.
- Pre-meal tests are the most useful, as post-meal tests will rise according to type of food eaten.
- A post-meal test can be useful in noting the effects of foods eaten.
- Blood tests should be carried out more frequently during the course of an infection or intercurrent illness (2-4 hourly).
- Should blood glucose levels be consistently high or low, reasons for this should be examined and appropriate action taken.
- Occasional high tests should not be acted upon unless they consistently occur at the same time of day.
- Should lifestyle be different on weekdays or weekends, blood tests will demonstrate this. Adjustments in food, medication or insulin may be required.
- If extra activity or exercise are anticipated, blood glucose levels should be checked beforehand and extra carbohydrate taken or insulin reduced (or both).

- Following extra activity or exercise, blood glucose levels should be checked soon afterwards and some hours later (in case of delayed hypoglycaemia).
- Correctly *taught* and *timed* visually read blood testing strips are a sufficient guide to blood glucose levels.
- If the person with diabetes has poor vision or is colour blind, blood glucose meters (for use with their appropriate strips) are available for purchase (or loan from hospital clinics or centres), providing a numerical reading.
- Strip guides (for guiding blood onto the test patch) and talking meters are available for those who are blind.
- *Meters should only be suggested in association with education regarding their use.*
- *Correct meter care and quality control are essential* where meters are used for self-monitoring (as well as those used in a surgery).
- Blood monitoring strips are available on prescription (free – except for people treated with diet alone, under the ages of 60 and 65 years of age – women and men respectively).
- Finger pricking devices may be obtained by prescription from hospital clinics or centres. Alternatively they can be purchased by the individual. They are not available on FP10.
- Recording of blood tests should be taught and a testing diary provided (available free – see resources list Chapter 16). These may also be obtained from the hospital clinic or centre.

Note Should there be any problems regarding self-monitoring using blood tests, interpretation of results, action to be taken or a blood glucose meter required, it is advisable to refer the person concerned to the local hospital clinic or diabetes centre.

11 Eye care and screening

At annual review and if necessary more frequently, the primary care team should be concerned with eye care as an essential part of diabetes care and surveillance.

Eye care for people with diabetes attending the hospital

A member of the primary care team should check annually (from people with diabetes attending surgery or from hospital letters held in the general practice records) for the following:

* That visual acuity has been checked.
* That both eyes have been screened for diabetic retinopathy (through dilated pupils).
* That action has been taken (if appropriate) following the detection of any visual problems.
* That a visit has been made (annually) to an optician for optical tests and sight correction (if required).

Eye care for people with diabetes attending the practice

Eye care for people with diabetes attending the practice should be provided for the following:

* People with diabetes solely attending the practice for their care.
* People attending the practice, where care is 'shared', and eye care has not been provided by the hospital.
* People who are housebound and cannot attend hospital or practice for eye care.

What eye care should be provided by the primary care team?

* Visual acuity (checked annually).

- Check that optician is being visited annually.
- Fundoscopy (with dilated pupils) for the detection of diabetic retinopathy (annually).
- Information about laser therapy.
- Appropriate and timely referral to an ophthalmologist.

Visual acuity

- Visual acuity is a simple test indicating the acuteness of central vision for distance and near or reading vision.
- In the condition of diabetes, *normal* visual acuity may be shown, even though diabetic retinopathy is demonstrated by fundoscopy.
- The testing of visual acuity in people with diabetes is necessary because normal to good vision is required for the following reasons:
  a) Checking monitoring strips
  b) Checking tablets taken (type and dose)
  c) Checking insulin given (type and dose)
  d) Inspecting feet
  e) Checking skin lesions (for infection)
  f) Checking injection sites
  g) Reading instructions/educational material

- Visual acuity should be checked annually and followed up by a fundoscopy examination through dilated pupils.
- If pupils are dilated before visual acuity is checked, the patient will be *unable* to see the test chart.
- If visual acuity has deteriorated and no diabetic retinopathy is detected by fundoscopy, the person with diabetes should be advised to visit an ophthalmic optician for optical tests and sight correction if required.
- Sight deterioration may be due to cataract which (if mature) requires referral to an ophthalmologist for removal (both eyes may be affected by cataract).
- If diabetic retinopathy is detected and is sight threatening, urgent referral to an ophthalmologist is required.
- During stabilisation of diabetes (following diagnosis or where medication or insulin have been introduced or adjusted), visual disturbances, such as blurred vision, may be experienced. These visual changes may vary from individual to individual and will improve in time.
- Possible visual changes such as these should be explained (they occur due to changes in glucose levels in the lens of the eye).
- The person concerned should be reassured and told that once blood glucose levels settle, vision will improve.

- On diagnosis and if alterations in therapy are made (such as a change from medication to insulin), the person concerned should be advised not to visit an optician until visual changes have settled (this may be a period of two to three months).
- Considerable inconvenience and expense (if new spectacles are advised) will be incurred by the person with diabetes if they are not correctly informed of the possibility of visual changes.

Note Annual eye tests (by an optician) are *free* for people with diabetes.

Equipment required for testing visual acuity

Snellen chart
- There are two sizes of chart (printed on black on a white ground).
- Pictorial charts are available for those unable to read letters.

Six metre chart
- The chart is placed at adult eye level 6 metres (20 feet) from the spot where the patient will stand to view the chart (the 6 metres should be measured and the standing spot marked on the floor with adhesive tape).
- The 6 metre chart can be used in a small space (the chart placed at 3 metres [10 feet] behind the standing spot) with the patient viewing the chart through a mirror 3 metres (10 feet) in front of the patient.

Three metre chart
- A 3 metre chart can be used where only a small space is available (eg in a small surgery).
- The three metre chart should not be used with a mirror.

Lighting
- Whichever size test chart is used, the chart should be well lit.
- A suitably placed angled lamp may be required.

Plain card
- Necessary to cover eye not being tested (hand not satisfactory).

'Pinhole' card
- Used to exclude errors of refraction.
- Provided free by some pharmaceutical companies (eg Wellcome).
- Card can be improvised by cutting out a square piece of card 10 cm (4") x 10 cm (4") and inserting a hole in the centre 1 mm in diameter using a needle (see Fig 11.1).

Fig 11.1 'Pinhole' card.

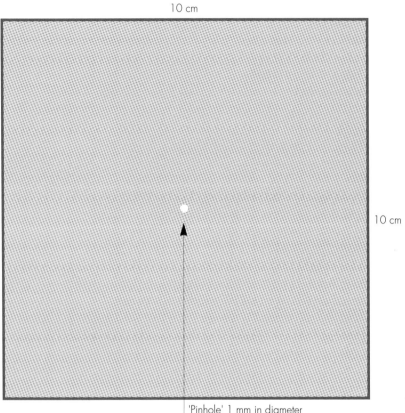

10 cm

10 cm

'Pinhole' 1 mm in diameter

- The 'pinhole' card should be held 3-7 cm (1-2") in front of the eye being tested.

Near vision test cards
- Near vision test cards are available, although usually used in an ophthalmic department or by an optician.
- The cards consist of different sizes of printer's type, each size being numbered.
- The near vision is tested in each eye and recorded.
- If the patient uses reading glasses, these should be worn during the test.
- The test cards should be well lit and held at a comfortable distance (approximately 25 cm (10") from the eyes).
- The near vision is recorded as the card number of the smallest printer's type that can easily be read.

Colour vision test cards
- Colour vision test cards are usually in book form.
- The books of cards show colours in mosaic patterns and are designed to test different types of colour vision defects.
- Colour vision test books may be used in the practice to detect defects which may be important for driving, employment and for detecting colour changes in monitoring test strips.

To test distance vision

- Distance vision is tested at 6 metres (20 feet) as rays of light at this distance are parallel.
- If the patient wears spectacles constantly, vision should be recorded with and without spectacles (if the vision does not show improvement with spectacles, this may be due to incorrect spectacle prescription, cataracts, diabetic retinopathy or other retinal defect).
- Each eye should be tested and recorded separately. The eye not being tested should be covered by a hand held card.
- Visual acuity is expressed as a fraction and abbreviated as VA on the diabetes or GP record.
- The *numerator* is the distance in metres at which the person can read a particular line of letters on the chart.
- The *denominator* is the distance at which a person with average vision can read the same line, eg if the seventh line is read at a distance of 6 metres, this is shown as VA 6/6.
- If some letters in the line are read, but not all, the result is expressed as VA 6/6-2 (ie 2 letters incorrect at 6/6). See Fig11.2.
- For deteriorating vision (less than 6/60), the distance between the patient and the chart is reduced a metre at a time and the vision recorded as 5/60, 4/60, 3/60, 2/60, 1/60).
- Counting fingers (VA=CF) may be used if the patient cannot read the top letter at a distance of 1 metre.
- For vision reduced even further, the hand is moved in front of the eye(s) at 30 cm (VA=HM). (HM=hand movements only.)
- If vision has deteriorated (and is not improved by spectacles), the 'pinhole' card should be used to detect errors of refraction.
- If visual acuity is improved using a pinhole card, visual deterioration is due to poor focusing. An optician's assessment is required and corrective action taken.
- If visual acuity is not improved (with spectacles or with a pinhole card), some other cause for the deterioration must be looked for.

Fig 11.2 Examples of visual acuity.

```
                                                    TEST CHART
                                                        T
                                                       60
                                                       X U
Example 1                                              36
At 6 metres, the patient can only read D Z A  ————————— D  Z  A
Record as 6/24  ——————————————————————————————————————— 24
                                                     P  W  F  H
Example 2                                               18
At 6 metres, the patient can only read V Z T D X ————— V  Z  T  D  X
Record as 6/12  ——————————————————————————————————————— 12
                                                   N  A  F  T  E  L
Example 3                                               9
At 6 metres, the patient can read A T X P N ———————— A  U  T  X  P  Z  N
Record as 6/6-2  —————————————————————————————————————— 6
                                                 F  O  N  T  U  M  P  X
                                                        5
                                                 Z  A  K  H  T  P  N  D  F
                                                        4
                                             H  D  A  Z  U  X  T  F  N  P
```

Testing for visual acuity – step by step

1. Explain to the patient the reasons for the test and how it will be carried out.

2. Place the patient (on the marked standing spot) facing the chart at the appropriate distance (depending on the chart size or, in a small space, where a mirror is used).

3. a) If the patient does not wear spectacles, ask him/her to cover the LEFT eye with a plain card.

b) If the patient does wear spectacles for distance vision, ask him/her to retain them and cover the LEFT eye with a plain card.

c) Always test the RIGHT eye first (to facilitate recording and avoid confusion). See Fig 11.3.

d) Always record whether spectacles/'pinhole' are used (see Fig 11.3). For example:

cum	= c	=	with (spectacles)
sine	= s	=	without (spectacles)
'pinhole'	= ph	=	'pinhole' card used.

Fig 11.3 Recording visual acuity (example).

R	VA	L
6/24	s	6/9
6/9	c	6/6
6/6	ph	6/6

- Visual acuity should be recorded annually.
- Records can be compared from year to year.
- Deterioration of visual acuity should be brought to the attention of the doctor and a visit to an optician advised.

Opticians

There are three types of optician.

The dispensing optician

- The dispensing optician is available almost everywhere and can be found in many high streets.
- The dispensing optician tests sight, prescribes and provides spectacles according to the prescription.
- The dispensing optician does not detect other ophthalmic defects.

The contact lens fitter

- The contact lens fitter specialises in contact lens prescription and provision.
- The contact lens fitter tests sight, prescribes and provides contact lenses (and lens care advice/preparations).

Note Contact lenses can be used by people with diabetes. Soft contact lenses are generally advised.

The ophthalmic optician

- The ophthalmic optician is available almost everywhere.
- The ophthalmic optician tests sight, prescribes and provides spectacles according to the prescription.
- The ophthalmic optician can test for other eye problems, eg raised intra-ocular pressure (glaucoma).

- The ophthalmic optician can detect other defects including diabetic retinopathy
- Ophthalmic opticians are used by many general practitioners to screen for diabetic retinopathy. If retinopathy is detected by the optician a 'green card' with a record of the optician's examination is sent to the general practitioner, who then refers the patient to an ophthalmologist – if this is indicated.

Note Although experienced practitioners at ophthalmoscopy, ophthalmic opticians screening for diabetic retinopathy do not always dilate pupils prior to fundoscopy examination. Dilatation of the pupils (by instillation of mydriatic drops) is essential for the detection of diabetic retinopathy – particularly peripheral maculopathy (retinopathy detected at the periphery of the retinal fundus and not uncommon in people with non-insulin dependent diabetes of long duration. This may also be present at diagnosis).

Fundoscopy

Equipment

1. A darkened room.
2. An approved ophthalmoscope with good batteries.
3. Mydriatic drops (Tropicamide 0.5% or 1%). Tropicamide 1% may be necessary (particularly for people with dark brown irises).
4. Tissues.

Preparation of patient

- The patient should be pre-warned of fundoscopy examination and if necessary accompanied (particularly if elderly).
- Short distance vision is affected by the mydriatic drops (effect 2-4 hours), although blurring of vision may be experienced for up to 24 hours.
- Mydriatic drops do not preclude driving, although it may be prudent for the patient to avoid this.
- Mydriatic drops do not require reversal.
- Darkened glasses should be worn (following mydriatic drops) in bright sunlight.

   Prior to pupil dilatation and fundoscopy examination, the following history should be taken:
- General medical history.
- Diabetes history (type, duration, treatment)

- History of eye problems (hereditary eye disease, cataracts, chronic glaucoma etc) and any eye surgery or treatment undergone or in progress.
- Any visual symptoms experienced.
- Visual acuity (unaided or with distance glasses, with or without 'pinhole' card).
- Examination of both eyes (for cataract, iritis rubeosis).

!Warning!
- If the patient has a lens implant in place following a cataract extraction, mydriatic drops should NOT be used.
- Mydriatic drops can precipitate closed angle glaucoma in patients with shallow anterior chambers. The onset is rapid and painful. The eye becomes red with a hazy cornea and blurred vision. This is however, very rare. Should it occur, immediate ophthalmic treatment is required.
- The possibility of precipitation of acute glaucoma should not preclude the use of mydriatic drops and fundoscopy examination, as this complication is so rare and, in the practice situation, can be quickly referred for treatment.
- It is important that the retinas are screened annually for diabetic retinopathy.

Chronic glaucoma
- Chronic glaucoma (as well as cataract) is more common in people with diabetes.
- The development of chronic glaucoma is slow and painless.
- It is important that intra-ocular pressure is measured and recorded annually.
- The measurement of intra-ocular pressure may be carried out in general practice (with appropriate equipment), by an ophthalmic optician or in screening programmes carried out by hospital ophthalmic departments.
- People with diabetes and individuals (aged 40 years and over) who are close relatives to known glaucoma patients are eligible for FREE NHS tests for the detection of glaucoma.
- Chronic glaucoma results in a gradual reduction in the peripheral field of vision, so insidious that the patient is unaware, even at a late stage, when tunnel vision develops.
- Treatment consists of eye drops or oral agents. If these fail, surgical trabeculectomy or laser therapy is carried out.

Fundoscopy examination – step by step

Instilling mydriatic drops
- Explain procedure to patient.
- Warn patient that drops will sting for a few moments.
- Sit patient in chair with head back.

- Stand behind patient and ask him/her to look up.
- Pull down lower eyelid and allow drop to fall into lower fornix.
- The eye will close in a reflex action.
- Mop with tissues.
- Repeat in other eye.
- Keep patient seated in darkened room for 15-20 minutes (to allow pupils to dilate as fully as possible).
- If pupils do not dilate sufficiently following the above procedure, a further drop in each eye may be necessary.

Following fundoscopy examination by doctor
- Record results.
- Check vision is satisfactory (this may be blurred).
- Check transport/availability of accompanying person (particularly if patient is elderly) before allowing home.

If diabetic retinopathy is detected
- The patient should be informed.
- Information should be given as to the extent of retinal damage.
- If the retinopathy is sight threatening, immediate referral should be made to an ophthalmologist.
- A great deal of reassurance and support are required because of the fear surrounding possible visual loss and the fear of eye treatment (laser therapy or surgery).
- Detailed explanations regarding the degree of retinal damage (following possible further tests – such as retinal photography) and a plan of treatment will be given by the ophthalmologist.
- Information regarding laser therapy for patients is provided (see Fig 11.4).

Fig 11.4 Laser therapy: patient information sheet.

- The laser is a machine which produces a small spot of very bright light.
- The light is so bright it produces a burn wherever it is focused.
- The lasers used produce blue-green or occasionally red light.
- Although the laser makes a burn in your eye, it is not usually painful because the back of your eye (the retina) cannot feel pain.
- Sometimes, however, if you have had a lot of laser treatment, it may be painful and you will be offered a local anaesthetic.
- Laser treatment is almost always done in an out-patient department.
- You will be perfectly fit to go home after the treatment.
- Your vision may be blurred or you may be dazzled by bright light (take dark glasses with you).
- You should not drive home afterwards.
- It is best to be accompanied to the laser clinic.
- After the treatment, you may notice some reduction in your sight. This usually only lasts a short time and only occasionally as much as a week. Occasionally you may experience headaches.
- As only one eye is treated at a time, if your other eye sees well, your vision should not be too badly affected.
- Most people do not need to take time off work following treatment.
- If you declare on your driving license application form that you have had laser treatment (as you are required to do), it is likely that you will have to have a visual fields test (to test the extent of your vision).
- If you have to have large amounts of laser treatment your field of vision may be affected.
- Provided that you can read a number plate at 25 metres (67 feet) with or without spectacles, and you pass the visual fields test (as most people do), there will be no problem about you driving.

References

MacKinnon, M (1991). *Visual Acuity.* Diabetic Nursing 2:9-10

Talbot, J F (1990). *Diabetes and your eyes.* Notes.

Vick, C L (1992). *Eye Screening in Diabetes Mellitus – a Non-Medical Review.* Treating Diabetes 8-11

12 Foot care and surveillance

At annual review and if identified as 'at risk' more frequently, the primary care team should be concerned with foot care as an essential part of diabetes care and surveillance.

Foot care

Foot care for people with diabetes attending the hospital

A member of the primary care team should check annually (from people with diabetes attending the surgery or from hospital letters held in the general practice records) for the following:

1. That feet have been examined.
2. That shoes have been examined.
3. That action has been taken (if appropriate) following the detection of foot problems or inappropriate footwear.
4. That education about foot care and shoes has been provided.

Foot care for people with diabetes attending the practice

Foot care for people with diabetes attending the practice should be provided for the following:

- People with diabetes solely attending the practice for their care.
- People attending the practice where care is 'shared' and foot care has not been provided by the hospital.
- People who are housebound and cannot attend hospital or practice for foot care.

What foot care should be provided by the primary care team?

1. Identification of people with diabetes 'at risk' of foot problems.
2. An annual examination of both feet (more often for those 'at risk').
3. An annual examination of shoes.
4. Education about foot care and footwear.

5. Appropriate and timely referral for chiropody treatment.

6. Appropriate and timely referral to a specialist foot clinic (if needed).

Feet at risk

The non-diabetic foot

It should be remembered that feet are at risk in the non-diabetic population under the following conditions:

The young person
- Ill-fitting footwear
- Poor quality footwear
- Trauma
- Congenital spine, hip, lower limb deformities
- In pregnant women – changing weight and gait

In middle age
- Foot deformities
- Ill-fitting footwear
- Poor quality footwear
- Increasing weight
- Changing gait

The elderly
- Poor vision
- Decreasing mobility
- Living alone
- Foot deformities
- Poor circulation
- Concurrent medical problems
- Ill-fitting footwear
- Poor quality footwear
- Changing weight
- Changing gait

The diabetic foot

The two major complications of diabetes, causing foot ulceration, are (see Fig 12.1):
- Abnormal circulation (micro- and macro-vascular disease – ischaemia)
- Diabetic neuropathy (autonomic and peripheral)

It is important to recognise that one or other or both of these complications may be present in the same patient and to be able to recognise the differences between them and the associated factors leading to foot ulceration.

Fig 12.1 The major complications of diabetes causing foot problems.

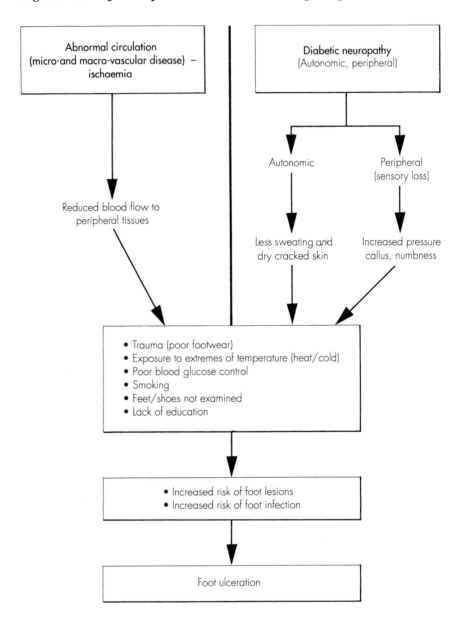

Fig 12.2 The ischaemic and neuropathic foot.

The ischaemic foot	The neuropathic foot
History **1**. Presence of intermittent claudication (calf pain) present when walking, relieved by rest.	*History* **1**. Corns, calluses and ulcers are usually painful.
2. Rest pain is a constant severe pain in toes, foot or calf, even thighs and buttocks, when severe.	**2**. Questioning may reveal that the patient is unaware of lesions or that they are not troublesome.
3. Pain occurs at rest and is aggravated when in sleeping position.	**3**. Enquire about general sensation (feeling in the legs and feet).
	4. A lack of feeling or 'pins and needles' or burning may be reported.
Examination *Colour:* Pale to cyanosed	*Examination* *Colour:* Normal to pink.
Temperature: Cold.	*Temperature:* Warm.
Pulses (Dorsalis Pedis Posterior Tibial) Diminished or absent.	*Pulses (Dorsalis Pedis Posterior Tibial)* Present or may be full and bounding.
Sensation: Present.	*Sensation:* Diminished or absent.
Knee/Ankle Jerk: Present.	*Knee/Ankle Jerk:* Diminished or absent.

Examination of the feet

Equipment required:

- Examination couch or foot stool (second chair).
- A good light source.
- Cotton wool (to test 'light' sensation).

- Neurotips (or a pin may be used – for 'sharp' sensation).
- Patella hammer (to test knee/ankle jerk).
- A 'C' tuning fork CO128 (to test vibration perception).
- Wound swab (accompanying laboratory form).

Note A Doppler ultrasound can be used for the measurement of blood flow and a biothesiometer can be used for the detection of diminished vibration perception. These two items of equipment are expensive and not essential.

The examination
1. Shoes, socks (tights or stockings) should be removed.
2. The patient should be examined lying on a couch or seated comfortably with both legs and feet raised (on a foot stool or second chair).
3. Both feet should be examined for the following:

- Condition of the skin (lower legs and feet).
- Check for dry, flaky skin.
- Check for cracks or evidence of fungal infection between each toe (athlete's foot).
- Check colour of skin (lower legs and feet).
- Check for corns, calluses, other deformities (particularly on pressure bearing points eg metatarsal heads).
- Check condition of toe nails (whether thickened, long or horny).
- Check nail cutting technique/in-growing toe nails.
- Check for discoloration/abnormal skin lesions.
- Check for evidence of infection – ie pain, lack of pain, numbness, inflammation, cellulitis or exudate (which may be purulent).
- Ensure that upper, lower surfaces of feet and toes (including heels) are carefully examined.

4. All abnormalities/changes should be recorded.
5. A doctor or further trained member of the primary care team should complete the examination of the feet for the following:

- Palpation of dorsalis pedis and posterior tibial pulses.
- If ischaemia is severe, pulses throughout the lower limb should be palpated.
- Changed, diminished or absent pulses should be recorded.
- Sensation testing – by checking light touch sensation, sharp/blunt discrimination and vibration perception.
- Testing for light touch, sharp/blunt discrimination and vibration perception should be carried out from toe to mid-calf region.
- For comparison, the stimulus should first be applied to the patient's

outstretched hand and then repeated on the lower limbs and feet – with the eyes closed.

- Testing for motor neuropathy should include examination for weakness or deformities in the toes and feet.
- In addition, knee and ankle jerks should be checked (with a patella/tendon hammer).
- Sensation defects should be recorded.
- Foot ulcers should be examined for inflammation and discharge (and a swab taken for bacterial analysis).
- Foot problems identified should be recorded and discussed with the patient as appropriate.

Examination of the shoes
Shoes should be examined inside and outside for:

- Evidence of wear and tear generally.
- The need for repair.
- Evidence of gait change (one shoe more worn than the other).
- Evidence of excessive weight bearing (heel on sole worn down).
- Evidence of perforation of soles or heels (by nails etc).
- Evidence of abrasive heels (especially with new shoes).
- Evidence of damaging projections inside the shoes (causing pressure).
- Evidence of worn insoles (causing pressure).
- Problems identified with shoes should be recorded and discussed with the patient.

Examination of socks/tights/stockings
Socks, tight or stocking should be examined for:

- Type of material (whether constricting – nylon or elasticated).
- Type of washing powder used (biological washing powders can be irritant).
- Method of holding up (eg garters should not be used).
- Presence and thickness of seams (these can cause traumatic ulcers).
- Problems identified should be recorded and discussed with the patient.

Identification of people at risk of diabetic foot problems

People with diabetes 'at risk' of foot problems should be identified and recorded on the diabetes register, and/or on the recall system – for more frequent follow up.

Those at risk are:
- People with peripheral vascular disease (ischaemia)
- People with neuropathy
- The elderly
- People with poor vision
- People unable to care for their own feet
- Those living alone
- Those with poor mobility/dexterity
- People with foot deformities
- People with a history of foot ulceration
- Those who are heavy smokers
- People with poor glycaemic control

Treatment

Foot care advice

- Advice about foot care should be individually given and reinforced as and when appropriate (at least annually).
- Foot care advice should preferably be provided for the relative/carer, as the person with diabetes (particularly if they are 'at risk') may be unable to follow the advice themselves.
- An individual leaflet may be supplied, written in the presence of the person with diabetes, relative or carer.
- Foot care information leaflets may be available locally or free from the British Diabetic Association or pharmaceutical companies (see resources list Chapter 16).
- Information and advice for patients about foot care, shoes and footwear (socks, stockings, tights) is given in Figs 12.4, 12.6 and 12.8.

Fig 12.3 Foot.

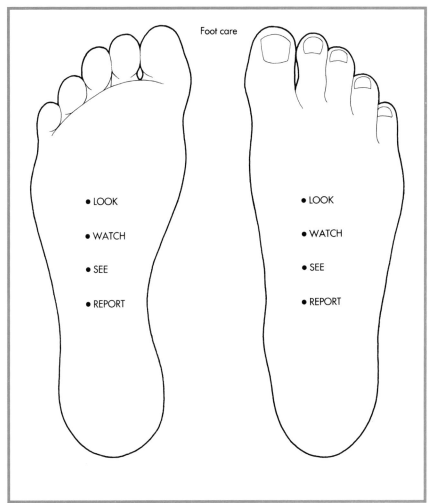

Foot care

- LOOK

- WATCH

- SEE

- REPORT

- LOOK

- WATCH

- SEE

- REPORT

12

Fig 12.4 Patient information: diabetes foot care advice.

10 points

- Inspect feet daily (If possible – use a mirror if you cannot reach your feet)

- Keep feet clean (Wash well, dry between toes)

- Avoid extremes of temperature – heat/cold
    - Avoid very hot baths (Put cold water in first then add hot water. Test with elbow)
    - Avoid hot fires/radiators
    - Avoid hot water bottles (Use an electric heat pad and check safety annually or alternatively wear warm bed socks)

- Report sores, skin damage **immediately** to your doctor

- Cut nails according to shape of toe

- If you cannot cut nails – go to State Registered Chiropodist

- Do not treat corns or calluses yourself – go to State Registered Chiropodist

- Do not use surgical blades or corn paring knives on your feet

- Keep skin moist (use hand cream, olive oil or E45 cream, available on prescription)

- Wear shoes or slippers at all times

Fig 12.5 Shoes.

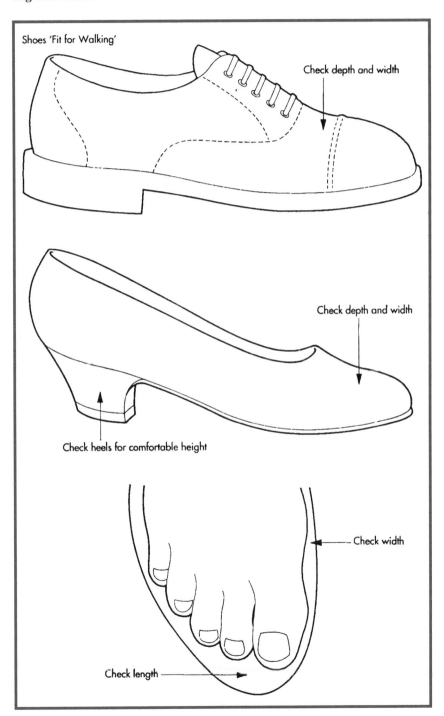

Shoes 'Fit for Walking'

Check depth and width

Check depth and width

Check heels for comfortable height

Check width

Check length

Fig 12.6 Patient information: diabetes care shoe advice.

10 points

- Feel inside and check the outside of your shoes before putting them on (check for ridges, sharp points or protruding nails)

- Buy shoes that fit well (depth, width and length, heels not too high – approximately 3-7 cm (1-2"))

- Go to a shoe shop that will measure and fit your shoes correctly

- Remember that shoes should be fitted individually (each foot is slightly different in shape and size)

- If the shape of your foot has altered you may need specially fitted insoles or shoes (these can be supplied by your chiropodist or shoe fitter)

- Do not wear new shoes for long (no more than 1-2 hours at a time)

- Newly fitted shoes should be slightly longer than your longest toe when you are standing – your foot lengthens when you walk (your toes should move freely inside your shoes)

- Make sure shoes are not too tight (watch out for creases when you walk)

- Make sure shoes are not too loose (watch out for your feet sliding or heels/toes rubbing)

- Do not wear rubber boots for too long. Do not wear 'work' boots for too long (change into shoes as soon as you can)

Fig 12.7 Socks/stockings/tights.

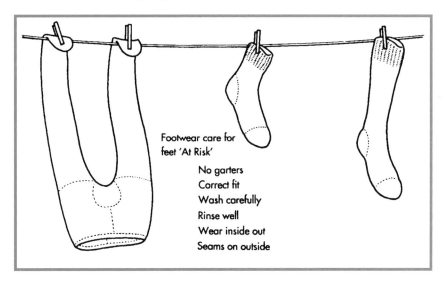

Footwear care for
feet 'At Risk'

No garters
Correct fit
Wash carefully
Rinse well
Wear inside out
Seams on outside

Fig 12.8 Patient information: diabetes care – footwear advice (socks, stockings, tights).

8 points

- If possible, change socks, stockings or tights daily
- Wear the correct size.
- Socks should be of natural fibres (wool or cotton) and loose fitting
- Do not wear garters
- Wash in non-irritant detergent (eg non-biological washing powder) and rinse well
- If you have poor circulation or nerve damage, wear socks, stockings or tights inside out (so that the seams are on the outside of your foot)
- Repair damaged socks, stockings, tights or discard and use new ones
- If you have varicose veins, requiring support stockings – seek medical advice (for the correct type and size of stocking when you obtain your prescription)

Treatment of diabetic foot ulcers by the primary care team

If foot ulcers are reported to, or detected by, the primary care team, the following procedure should be carried out:
- Both feet should be examined
- Glycaemic control should be reviewed
- A wound swab should be taken (if appropriate)
- If infection is present, antibiotics should be prescribed (these may be required long term)
- The foot, lower limb should be rested whenever possible
- When resting – the foot, lower limb should be elevated (at least to hip level)
- Light non-adherent dressings should be used
- Elastoplast should NEVER be used on the skin
- Constricting (elastic) bandages should not be used
- Both feet should be examined regularly
- If infection persists, the ulcer does not heal or glycaemic control is poor, referral to a diabetes foot clinic (or the hospital diabetes team) should be made.

Criteria for referral to specialist foot clinic or hospital diabetes team

Referral should be made for the following reasons:

- The presence of a non-healing foot ulcer
- Severe ischaemia
- Autonomic or peripheral neuropathy causing sensory loss
- Pain/numbness in feet lower limbs
- Poor 'glycaemic' control in those identified 'at risk' of foot problems
- Those with a history of foot ulceration
- People with a foot deformity (which may be caused by neuropathy)
- Where osteomyelitis is suspected (an x-ray is required to confirm this)
- People requiring 'custom made' insoles or special shoes
- People identified 'at risk' requiring regular chiropody and surveillance (outside the scope of the primary care team)

Criteria for referral to a State Registered Chiropodist

Referral should be made for the following reasons:

- Where toe nails cannot be cut by the person with diabetes (due to visual impairment etc)
- Where toe nails cannot be cut by the relative or carer
- Where corns, calluses require treatment
- Where insoles or special shoes may be required
- Where general foot care/footwear advice is needed
- Where urgent chiropodist treatment is required
- Where an assessment is needed
- Where regular surveillance is required

References

British Diabetic Association (1993). *Non-insulin dependent diabetes Balance for Beginners.* 44-46

Woodburn J, Thomson C (1991). *The Diabetic Foot* 1991. Diabetic Nursing Vol 2; No 2:3-5

12

13 Education for self-management

Living with diabetes requires knowledge and experience, built up over time. The level and pace of learning varies greatly between individuals. It is important for health care professionals to appreciate the gaps between 'learning', 'understanding' and 'doing' and why such gaps occur.

Reasons for 'learning', 'understanding', and 'doing' gaps

The newly diagnosed person
Considerable shock often accompanies the newly diagnosed person with diabetes. A sense of bereavement is felt, caused by the loss of health and fear of the unknown or of the future. This sense of shock and fear may also be felt by relatives and have a considerable impact on a whole family. It is at this time that a great deal of information may be passed to the person concerned, much of which is unnecessary at this stage and may even be counterproductive and confusing.

Preconceived ideas
Experiences of diabetes previously learned from family members or friends may have been negative and even horrific, resulting in extreme fear and concern. This may block any constructive discussion regarding self-management at an early stage.

Fear of living with diabetes
Preconceived ideas may lead to particular concerns of living with diabetes, such as restrictions in eating, drinking and everyday activities. Worries may be expressed regarding employment, driving, travel, holidays and, in younger people, the implications of diabetes on college, leaving home, starting work and starting a family.

Culture
Culture and personal health beliefs have a considerable bearing on attitudes to disease and coping with a life long progressive condition, such as diabetes. In

certain societies, being overweight in a woman is regarded as beautiful and desir-able, in others the opposite is true. The diagnosis of diabetes in some culture may place the person concerned into a 'sick role', rendering the concept of living a healthy life with diabetes difficult to grasp.

Fear of long term complications of diabetes
Again preconceived ideas and some previous knowledge of diabetes may result in extreme concern (even a morbid fear) of complications, particularly regarding eyes and blindness, feet and amputation.

Physical difficulties
Elderly people in particular may have problems with physical disability and suf-fer a reduction in their mobility. The sight, hearing and senses of touch, smell and taste may become less acute with age.

Mental difficulties
People with mental handicap, illness or disability require particular care in their management. Much of the burden of their diabetes and concerns over its progres-sion will fall to relatives or carers, who require special support.

The ageing process affects the memory as well as the ability to take in infor-mation and act on it. As people become older, they may appear to cope quite well with living with diabetes but be reluctant to change certain habits built up over a lifetime.

13

Literacy and education
Literacy is assumed, both in our own society and in others. An illiterate person should not be deemed stupid, in fact the reverse may be true. Compensation by the person for illiteracy may be such that the problem is effectively disguised.

Educational levels, particularly regarding how the body works, should not be taken for granted. A highly intelligent and well educated person is often assumed to be knowledgeable and coping when, in fact, the diagnosis may be denied or fear of complications may lead to obsessional monitoring and control of blood glucose levels ruling the person's life.

Language
Language is obviously a barrier to communication where English is not the mother tongue. It is important that appropriate translation methods are used, such as help from family members if appropriate, health link workers or a telephone translation scheme such as Language Line (available in some health districts). Contact with local ethnic minority groups may also generate local interest in diabetes, translating expertise and materials into the appropriate language.

The greatest difficulty with language used by health care professionals is the use of medical terminology which is either not understood or misunderstood and, in most instances, is inappropriate. Most people are grateful for a simple non-technical explanation and will enquire further if this is insufficient.

Attitude

An attitude is describe as a 'settled mode of thinking and behaviour'. In diabetes, this is governed by what happens at diagnosis and immediately thereafter. Good management at this stage will set the scene for the future attitude towards diabetes and self-care. Positive ongoing support, that is non-judgmental and responsive to concerns expressed by the person with diabetes, will help to reinforce the person's desire to look after him/her self.

Information giving

There are six main problems of information giving as identified by people with diabetes. These are:

- *Incorrect information* – where facts given about diabetes are wrong. It is much better for the health care professional to admit ignorance and offer to find out the correct information.
- *Inconsistent information* – where several health care professionals are involved and different educational messages are received, giving a confusing picture.
- *Too much information* – where too many messages are given, often at the same time, particularly at or near the diagnosis.
- *Too little information* – where the information supplied or requested is insufficient for the person concerned to find it useful or helpful.
- *Inappropriate information* – where the information given is not appropriate to the diabetes requirements or the age and lifestyle of the person concerned.
- *Lack of up to date information* – where information is given at diagnosis or when specifically requested and no further or new information is offered. In order to avoid this, individual or group education programmes should be planned, recorded and new information offered as soon as it is learned by the doctor, nurse or other health care professional involved. One of the main reasons for this is the lack of continuing education by heath care professionals.

Home, work and social life

Home, work and social life influence the control and even the progression of diabetes. Unemployment, financial concerns and loneliness may be hidden, but may be the reason for a change in eating habits, shoes of a poorer quality, disinterest or depression.

Opportunities in careers, employment, in sport and other common life experiences may be over shadowed by the stigma of diabetes.

Lifestyle changes
Leaving home for the first time, a change of home or job, retirement or the loss of a partner may cause a major change in attitude and behaviour. Extra support and further education may be needed at these times.

Assessment for diabetes self-management and education

This should take place at annual review and if appropriate at every routine review. The assessment (by enquiry) should include:

- Demographic information/changes
- Family status/changes
- Employment status/changes
- Medical history/changes
- Lifestyle history/changes
- Diabetes management/changes

In addition, at diagnosis, (or for a person with diabetes who has recently joined the practice), the assessment (by enquiry or observation) should include the following:

- Family history of diabetes
- Preconceived ideas of diabetes
- Knowledge of diabetes/complications
- Circumstances surrounding diagnosis
- Feelings surrounding diagnosis (patient)
- Feelings surrounding diagnosis (family/carers)
- Culture/language
- Physical difficulties
- Mental difficulties
- Literacy/education
- Attitude to diabetes

Getting the message across

Initially, education about diabetes in the general practice situation is best provided individually following assessment, although it can be helpful for a person newly diagnosed to meet another person who has had the condition for a time and has come to terms with it. In association with information provided, the practice should be able to offer the following resources (see resources list Chapter 16).

- Titles of books/a book loan scheme
- Booklets, leaflets (available from pharmaceutical companies or the BDA)
- Address/telephone number – British Diabetic Association
- Address/telephone number – local branch, British Diabetic Association
- Local information regarding diabetes care and associated services (dietetics/chiropody)
- Supportive agencies
- Social services

Whenever possible, education provided should be backed up with written information or the help to obtain it.

Once the service for people with diabetes is established in the practice, group education sessions may prove valuable, the people with diabetes bringing along a relative or friend.

Group sessions for 8-10 people (more than this may be too inhibiting) can be held around a cup of tea or appropriate snack lunch (financed by sponsorship from an appropriate pharmaceutical company, if practice policy supports this).

Group diabetes education in the practice

Organisation
- Selecting group to be invited (ie people treated with diet, tablets or insulin)
- Selecting members of the primary care team to be involved (and group facilitator)
- Deciding time, length and place of session
- Arranging tea/coffee/snacks
- Setting objectives for the session (to be agreed by participants)
- Inviting participants (with a minimum of two weeks notice – see Fig 13.1.)
- Designing a simple evaluation form for participants to complete following the session (see Fig 13.2)

Invitations can be given verbally to people attending the diabetes clinic if the group session is planned well ahead (to save telephone calls/stamps) Alternatively, a letter of invitation may be sent (see Fig 13.1).

Fig 13.1 Sample letter of invitation for a group diabetes session.

Practice Telephone No.: 222333
The Medical Practice
Woolley End Road
Airedale Edge
SHEFFIELD
South Yorkshire

January 1994

Mrs P Johnson
The Tannery
Black Terrace
SHEFFIELD

Dear Mrs Johnson

Re: Diabetes Care

We are planning to hold a lunchtime session for people with diabetes to discuss:

- Planning meals
- Testing for sugar
- Other topics, as required

on Wednesday 14 February 1994, at 12.30 pm

The session will finish at 2 pm and a snack lunch will be provided.

You and your husband are warmly invited to attend. If you are unable to come, we would be grateful if you would let us know.

Yours sincerely

Dr A Smith (General Practitioner)   Mrs M Jones (Practice Nurse)

13

Fig 13.2 Sample evaluation form for use following a group diabetes session.

The Medical Practice
Woolley End Road
Airedale Edge
SHEFFIELD
South Yorkshire

Diabetes care – group session

Date:

In order to assess today's session, we would be grateful if you will fill in this form. Thank you.

Please delete the answer that does not apply to you and make your own comments.

1. Are you A person with diabetes?

A relative?

A friend?

2. Did you receive sufficient notice to attend today's session?

YES/NO

3. Meal planning

a) Was the topic covered sufficiently for you?

YES/NO

b) Were there aspects of the topic not covered?

YES/NO

c) What aspects of this topic would you have like discussed further? Please write them down:

4. Testing for sugar

a) Was the topic covered enough for you?

YES/NO

b) Were there aspects of the topic not covered?

YES/NO

c) What aspects of this topic would you have like discussed further? Please write them down:

5. What other topics discussed did you find useful in the session? Please write them down:

_____

_____

_____

_____

6. Did you find today's session helped you to understand more about living with diabetes?

YES/NO

7. Would you be interested in attending further group sessions relating to diabetes care?

YES/NO

8. Do you have any suggestions for future sessions? Please write them down:

_____

_____

_____

_____

Thank you for filling in this form.

Facilitating the session includes:
- Preparation of room
- Greeting participants
- Domestic arrangements (coats/toilets etc)
- Introductions
- Arrangements for tea/coffee/snacks
- Stating the aims of the session and discussing these with participants
- Identifying topics requested by participants
- Introducing topics
- Allowing discussion to progress around topics
- Time keeping
- Summarising session
- Organising evaluation form to be completed
- Arranging follow up/further session
- Dealing with any personal problems identified during the session
- Supervising departure of participants
- Clearing up
- Discussing evaluation forms and session with other members of the team
- Recording education session in practice and patient records

'Getting the message across' in diabetes education, whether to individuals or groups involves the following:

- Discussing and planning education concerned with the person with diabetes/relative/carer
- Listening
- Hearing what is being said
- 'Picking up' hidden worries and difficulties
- Responding to questions
- Dealing with urgent problems
- Asking the right questions in the right way
- Being non-judgmental
- 'Staging' information
- Providing small pieces of information at one time
- Obtaining feedback on information given
- Summarising information given
- Demonstrating practical skills
- Observing practical skills learned
- Being positive, encouraging and supportive
- Recording information given and skills learned
- Discussing and planning further education with the person with diabetes/relative/carer.

14 Living with diabetes: information requirements

These are 'key' points only, providing a focus for discussion. The information should be 'staged' to the appropriate time, or provided when questions are asked. Information given *must* be recorded (for legal reasons).

Following confirmation of diagnosis

Understanding diabetes

- Preconceived ideas/fear of complications
- Causes
- Symptoms
- Treatment/effect of treatment/benefits
- Preconceived ideas – living with diabetes

Dietary advice

- 'Diabetic foods' not necessary
- Assessment of food/meals (family)
- Targets for weight control (personal)
- Dietary changes required/discussed
- Meal planning (family)
- Contact/referral – dietitian

Care provision (where, how and who?)

- In general practice
- In hospital diabetes clinic
- Shared by general practice and hospital diabetes clinic
- Care provided in specialist clinics (eyes/feet)
- Changes in care provision
- Importance of regular review
- Importance of annual review

Contact numbers

- Telephone number of general practice/hospital diabetes services
- Use of contact numbers, if problems
- Use of contact numbers, if unwell

Living with diabetes (further information – as appropriate)

Medication (oral hypoglycaemic agents)

- Name of drug
- Reason for use of drug
- Effect of drug
- Side-effects of drug
- Dose of drug
- When to take drug
- Hypoglycaemic risk of drug (if a sulphonylurea)
- Symptoms of hypoglycaemia
- Prevention of hypoglycaemia
- Treatment of hypoglycaemia
- Continuation of drug supplies – ordering of prescription – notice required by practice
- Prescription exemption – DOH Form No P11 – signed by doctor – to FHSA

Insulin

- Name, type, dose, effect of insulin
- Giving the injection (how, where and when)
- Spare insulin (in fridge)
- Care and disposal of syringes, needles, pens
- Risk of hypoglycaemia
- Symptoms of hypoglycaemia
- Prevention of hypoglycaemia (carriage of glucose, identification)
- Treatment of hypoglycaemia (Hypostop/glucagon)
- Contact number to ring – if problems; diabetes nurse specialist/clinic/centre
- Insulin dose adjustments (when and how)
- Continuation of insulin and supplies – ordering of prescription – notice required by practice
- Prescription exemption – DOH Form No P11 – signed by doctor – to FHSA

Hyperglycaemia

- Symptoms
- Prevention
- Action to take

Other medication taken (eg steroids)

- Effect on diabetes control
- Action to take if control affected (eg seek advice from doctor)

Illness rules

- Continue with medication
- Drink plenty of liquid (tea, water)
- Test urine/blood 2-4 hourly
- If vomiting or illness persists CONTACT DOCTOR

Urine testing

- Reasons for testing (benefits)
- Demonstration of test strips
- How to test
- When to test and how often
- The meaning of the test in relation to blood glucose levels (of the individual)
- The renal threshold
- Recording tests
- Action to take if urine glucose levels high
- Prescription for strips (unless treated with diet alone)

Blood glucose monitoring

- Reasons for testing (benefits)
- Demonstration of test strips
- Demonstration of equipment for testing
- How to test
- When to test
- Interpretation of test results
- Recording tests
- Action to take if blood glucose levels outside negotiated target range
- Prescription for strips

Alcohol

- Risk of hypoglycaemia (with insulin and sulphonylureas)
- Drinking guidelines (BDA recommendations)
- Dangers when driving (especially with added risk of hypoglycaemia)
- Risk of weight gain (and hyperglycaemia)

Smoking

- General risks of smoking
- Added risk of smoking and diabetes
- Encouragement/support to stop smoking
- Follow up support if smoking stopped

Blood pressure

- What blood pressure means
- Importance of annual blood pressure check
- Importance of blood pressure control in association with diabetes
- Value of weight reduction, salt restriction and increased exercise, if blood pressure raised
- Alcohol restriction and caffeine reduction may also be helpful before drug treatment is used
- If drugs for raised blood pressure are prescribed, it is important that they are taken regularly.
- Effect of hypertensive drugs.

Special occasions, celebrations, eating out

- Important that these are enjoyed
- Important to know to adjust insulin – for enjoyment!
- Blood glucose levels will be higher if more food or sweet foods are taken
- Urine tests/blood tests may demonstrate higher blood glucose levels
- Urine/blood glucose levels should settle in a day or two
- Alcohol may lower blood glucose levels

Annual review

Importance and reasons for annual review – opportunity for:
- Overview of general health/lifestyle
- Overview of diabetes and education
- Review of targets for weight, blood pressure and blood glucose levels (explain HbA_1)

- Review of laboratory results
- Medical examination
- Sight test
- Screening for diabetic retinopathy
- Examination of feet and shoes
- Urine checked for presence of protein

Eye care and screening

- Sight test
- Check annual visit to optician for free eye test. Importance of correct spectacles
- Pupils will be dilated before back of eyes are examined by doctor
- Each eye checked by doctor using ophthalmoscope
- Report any eye problems immediately (to practice)

Foot and shoe care

- Examine feet and shoes regularly (use a mirror if necessary)
- Look for sore areas or cracks, especially between the toes
- Report problems immediately (to practice)
- Keep feet clean (regular washing and careful drying)
- Keep toe nails trimmed (a chiropodist may be needed)
- Avoid extremes of heat/cold
- Make sure new shoes fit (length, width and depth)
- Make sure socks, stockings or tights fit
- Avoid garters

14

Chiropody (may be required)

- For toe nails to be trimmed
- For treatment of corn, callus
- For insoles or special shoes
- For regular care

Family planning advice

- Fertility is not impaired in diabetes except in the presence of severe renal disease
- Oral contraception is effective (1% failure rate)
- Oral contraceptives should not be used in women with diabetes in the following circumstances:

      Older women

      Overweight women

      Those with small or large vessel disease

      Those with a family history of vascular disease

      Smokers

- High dose combined oral contraceptives should not be used in women with a previous history of gestational diabetes or who have diabetes
- Low dose combined oral contraceptives may be used in the short term (with monitoring of blood glucose levels and blood pressure)
- Low dose prostagens may be used (they may not be so well tolerated or effective)
- Intra-uterine contraceptive devices can be used except in women with a history of acute pelvic infection or pelvic inflammatory disease
- Barrier methods and sterilisation can be offered to all women with diabetes
- Vasectomy can be offered to men with diabetes

Pre-conception

- Blood glucose levels should be well controlled three months prior to conception
- Pre-pregnancy counselling, education and support should be planned
- Early referral is necessary

Pregnancy

- Continuing support and surveillance by obstetric and diabetes teams are necessary throughout pregnancy and in the post-natal period.
- Early referral is recommended
- Dietary adjustments may be required during the establishment of breast feeding
- Protection should be provided against rubella during pregnancy

Hormone replacement therapy (HRT)

- HRT can and should be used in women with diabetes (oestrogens have a cardioprotective effect)
- Progestogens have an anti-insulin effect
- Blood glucose levels should be carefully monitored
- Insulin doses may need adjustment

Impotence

- Often a 'hidden' problem
- Common in men with a long history of diabetes
- May be the cause of marital difficulties
- Failure to gain an erection may be due to:
    Nerve damage
    Poor circulation
    Psychological factors
- Treatment is available and is offered following assessment for possible causes.
    Treatments currently considered/offered are:
    Counselling
    Vacuum devices
    Self-injection of Papaverine (into the penis)
    Penile implants
- Referral is recommended

Cervical screening

- Should be offered to women with diabetes

Breast screening

- Should be offered to women with diabetes

14

Tetanus immunisation

- Should be offered to people with diabetes

Influenza vaccination

- Influenza may upset diabetes control (particularly in the frail and elderly)
- Protection should be offered if not medically contraindicated
- Diabetes control may be upset following 'flu vaccination
- Extra monitoring is advisable
- Medication or insulin therapy may require temporary adjustment

Children and young people with diabetes

- Require special care and management
- Parents need support
- Should be referred appropriately on diagnosis

- May have particular problems at certain stages of childhood and development (eg change of school, onset of puberty), requiring extra support
- Diabetes control can deteriorate quickly (especially during an illness). Urgent admission to hospital may be required
- All immunisations should be offered to children and young people with diabetes
- As adult life approaches, support and counselling are required in association with higher education, employment, social pressures, driving and living away from home for the first time.

Employment

- Safety of the person with diabetes and safety of other people (in association with hypoglycaemia) must be considered
- People with diabetes (insulin treated) are not usually accepted for:
    The armed forces
    The police service
    The merchant navy
    The fire brigade
    The prison service
    Working at heights
    Deep sea diving
    Working on oil rigs
    Coal face working
    Truck or bus driving
- People with diabetes may not be employed as pilots, on the flight deck or in air traffic control
- Shift work can be accommodated with flexible insulin regimes
- Those treated with diet alone, or diet and medication can undertake any occupation (as the risk of hypoglycaemia is small)

Sport and leisure

- Safety of the person with diabetes and safety of others (in association with hypoglycaemia) must be considered
- Risk factors should always be taken into account by those treated with insulin
- An accompanying person is a sensible precaution
- A few sports apply restrictions to people with diabetes
- Extra food and/or an insulin dose reduction may be needed relating to degree of activity
- Extra food (if treated with medication) may be needed relating to degree of activity

- Possibility of delayed hypoglycaemia (following strenuous activity). This may occur *many* hours later
- Symptoms, prevention and treatment of hypoglycaemia in association with sport and leisure activities

Driving

Car driving licences
- Car driving licences can be held by people with diabetes
- The DVLC must be informed of the presence of diabetes and any treatment change (eg from diet alone to medication or medication to insulin). This is required by law. NB This information must be provided and recorded. The decision to follow this advice is the responsibility of the individual concerned
- Licences are renewed every one, two or three years depending on health (of people treated with medication or insulin)
- Licence renewal forms are sent automatically before the expiry date. There is no fee for renewal
- Licence renewal is granted following completion of the form (including signed consent for the individual's doctor to be consulted by the DVLC, if required) by the person with diabetes
- A medical check may be requested by the DVLC
- Those treated with diet alone are not subject to licence restrictions (for diabetes). They can retain their 'until aged 70' privilege
- The driver *must* inform his/her driving insurance company of the presence of diabetes
- Some insurance companies load the driver's premium. This should be challenged. Advice on sympathetic companies can be obtained from the British Diabetic Association

Vocational driving licences
- Vocational driving licences are required for Large Goods Vehicles (LGV) and Passenger Carrying Vehicles (PCV)
- People with diabetes, whose condition is treated with diet alone, or diet and medication and are well controlled may hold these licences
- People with diabetes treated with diet and insulin may NOT hold these licences (even if they held a licence prior to commencing insulin treatment). An exception to this rule is only made for those who have previously held a vocational licence issued by a licensing authority in the knowledge of their insulin treatment
- Holders of vocational driving licences must inform the DVLC on commencement of insulin treatment. NB This information must be provided and recorded.

The decision to follow this advice is the responsibility of the individual concerned.

- The licence will be revoked
- There is however a statutory right of appeal (details are sent from the DVLC when the licence is revoked)
- Advice regarding appeals against the withdrawal of car and vocational driving licences can be obtained from the British Diabetic Association
- People with visual impairment should not drive
- People who have lost their warning signs of hypoglycaemia should not drive
- Drivers should know the symptoms, prevention and treatment of hypoglycaemia
- Sweets/biscuits should always be available in the vehicle
- If hypoglycaemic warning signs occur the driver should:
    Move as safely as possible to the side of the road
    Stop the car and remove the keys from the ignition
    Move to the passenger seat and take sweets/biscuits
    Resume driving ONLY when safe to do so
    Have a substantial snack or meal as soon as possible

Life insurance policies

- As with motor insurance, life insurance is calculated according to age and state of health
- A life assurance policy already held should not be affected by the diagnosis of diabetes. It is not necessary to declare the diabetes
- If a new policy is taken out, the diabetes must be declared and the policy may be loaded. This can be challenged
- Advice about sympathetic insurance companies can be obtained from the British Diabetic Association

Note Professional guidance from brokers appointed by the British Diabetic Association may be obtained (see resources list Chapter 16).

Travel and holidays

- Immunisation and vaccination may be required. Exact details will depend on the country to be visited (available in the practice)
- Diabetes control may be temporarily affected (by immunisation)
- Travel insurance should include:
    Declaring diabetes (to obtain adequate cover)
    Checking extent of coverage
    Looking for a premium with a minimum coverage of £250,000
    Contacting British Diabetic Association for further information if required

- Obtain Form T1 (from local DSS office) – *The Travellers Guide to Health*
- Obtain Form E111 (from local DSS office) for medical care in EC countries
- The following should be considered prior to travel:

  Identification (card/bracelet)

  If travelling abroad, a doctors letter may be helpful when carrying
      syringes/insulin (particularly at customs points)

  Travel sickness prevention

  Anti-diarrhoea medication

  Anti-malarial medication (if appropriate)

  A supply of antibiotics

  Simple dressings

  Sufficient medication/insulin (insulin stored in a cool bag) and carried in
      hand luggage (U100 insulin is not available everywhere)

  Sufficient supplies of syringes/needle clipper (carried in hand luggage)

  Monitoring equipment (carried in hand luggage)

  Sunburn protection cream

  Sun hat

  Water purification tablets (if appropriate)

  Appropriate footwear

  Carriage of sweets/biscuits when travelling

  Contact British Diabetic Association for details about specific countries

The following organisations may also be helpful:

Thomas Cook Vaccination Centre
45 Berkeley Street
London W1A 1EB
Tel: 071 408-4157

British Airways Medical Services for Travellers Abroad
Tel: 071 831-5333

Hospital for Tropical Diseases Travel Clinic
180-2 Tottenham Court Road
London W1
Tel: 071 637-9899

Liverpool School of Tropical Medicine
Pembroke Place
Liverpool L3 5QA
Tel: 051 708-9393

Dental care

- Regular dental checks are important
- Dental infections may disturb diabetes control
- A painful mouth may prevent eating (particularly poorly fitting dentures) and a subsequent risk of hypoglycaemia
- There is no financial help for people with diabetes, relating to dental care

15 Monitoring and audit of practice diabetes care

The British Diabetic Association recommends these new audit guidelines for diabetes management in primary care.

Clinical audit and evaluation

Clinical audit of practice-based diabetes services should be performed regularly. The primary health care team should select which criteria they wish to audit and agree the standards of care against which to audit the quality of care provided. Medical Audit Advisory Groups (MAAGs) can also play an important role in facilitating clinical audit in primary care.

The accumulation of data at district, regional or national level, as recommended in the St Vincent Declaration, can enable the evaluation of the effectiveness of diabetes services in improving the health of people with diabetes.

The St Vincent Declaration specifies outcomes for which targets are set. Incidence rates for these outcomes are such that they can only be usefully interpreted at district, regional and national levels.

If data collected at practice level are to be aggregated, it is important to ensure standardisation of the data collected. A suggested minimum dataset for use in primary care is set out later in this chapter. The FHS Computer Unit is producing user requirements for Diabetes Care systems which will soon be available.

This process may be facilitated by the sending of information by practices to a district diabetes register for computer entry and analysis. Alternatively, if data is entered on practice computers, it should be in a format which can be analysed and amalgamated at district level.

As the outcomes for which targets are set in the St Vincent Declaration have long time scales, it is important to monitor measures of process, acute and intermediate outcomes and cardiovascular risk factors and other markers of late complications so that progress in the shorter term can also be monitored.

Process measures

- The level of ascertainment of patients with diagnosed diabetes.
- The apparent prevalence of diabetes in the practice population can be compared to the expected prevalence, taking into account the age and ethnic make-up of the practice population. A low figure may suggest under ascertainment.
- The proportion of identified patients reviewed within the last year.
- The proportion of identified patients in whom the following have been assessed within the last year:
    Body Mass Index
    Dietary intake – by state registered dietitian
    Tobacco consumption
    Urinalysis for proteinuria
    Blood pressure
    Glycosylated haemoglobin level (or fructosamine)
    Serum lipids
    Serum creatinine
    Eyes: visual acuity and fundoscopy through dilated pupils
    Feet: footwear, evidence of circulation problems and neuropathy
- The proportion of patients, identified as having the following problems, who are receiving appropriate management:
    Smoking
    Hypertension
    Hyperlipidaemia
    Eye problem
    Renal problem
    Foot problem

Outcome measures

Acute outcomes
- Proportion requiring hospital admission for ketoacidosis within last year
- Proportion requiring professional attention for hypo within last year
- Proportion of patients with cataract
- Proportion of patients with angina
- Proportion of patients with claudication
- Proportion of patients with symptomatic neuropathy
- Proportion of patients with impotence

Pregnancy outcomes
- Abortion rates in diabetic women: spontaneous miscarriages and terminations for congenital abnormality
- Still-birth and perinatal mortality rates amongst infants of diabetic mothers
- Incidence of congenital abnormalities

Intermediate outcomes
- Pattern of glycaemic control for each treatment group

Cardiovascular risk factors
- Proportion of patients who smoke
- Proportion of patients with hypertension
- Proportion of patients with raised cholesterol
- Proportion of patients with raised triglycerides

Markers of late complications
- Proportion of patients with proteinuria/microalbuminuria
- Proportion of patients with raised creatinine
- Proportion of patients with background and sight-threatening retinopathy
- Proportion of patients with absent foot pulses
- Proportion of patients with reduced vibration sense
- Proportion of patients with reduced pin-prick sensation
- Proportion of patients with foot ulceration

Late outcomes
- Proportion of patients who have had a myocardial infarction
- Proportion of patients who have had a stroke
- Proportion of patients with visual impairment
- Proportion of patients with severe visual impairment
- Proportion of patients with end-stage renal failure
- Proportion of patients who have had an amputation: below/above ankle
- Age-specific mortality rates in people with diabetes

15

Measures of health status, quality of life and patient satisfaction

- Psychological well-being
- Physical well-being
- Knowledge of diabetes
- Self-care performance
- Satisfaction with care
- Satisfaction with care delivery

Questionnaire surveys are required to monitor these measures. Attendance rates at clinic and waiting times to be seen in clinic can be used as proxy measures for patient satisfaction.

Recommended minimum dataset for management of diabetes in primary care

Patient details

Name	NHS Number	Date of Birth	Sex

Address

Year of diagnosis		Ethnic origin	

Annual review		Date performed	

History in		
last year of:	Admission for hyperglycaemia	
	Hypoglycaemia requiring professional attention	
	Angina/myocardial infarction	
	Transient ischaemic attack/stroke	
	Claudication/amputation: above or below ankle	
	Erectile impotence	

Procedures undertaken	Date performed	Result

Body mass index
Urinalysis for proteinuria/microalbuminuria
Blood pressure: systolic and diastolic
Tobacco consumption (cigarettes/day)
Glycosylated haemoglobin (or fructosamine)
Serum cholesterol and triglycerides
Serum creatinine
Visual acuity and ophthalmoscopy for cataract and retinopathy
Foot exam for pulses, vibration sensation and ulceration and general care

Diabetes therapy: insulin/oral hypoglycaemic agents/diet only

Hypertension and hyperlipidaemia therapy

Review by dietitian and/or chiropodist in last year

Routine follow-up:	GP only
	Shared care
	Hospital only

There are now a number of commercially available computer programmes. In addition the FHS Computer Unit of the Department of Health is also preparing a programme.

Family health services authority chronic disease management – Diabetes programme

In-year monitoring

Where general practices are providing a diabetes programme, an in-year monitoring report will be required by the Family Health Services Authority (FHSA). The following information will be requested:

- Any recent changes made to the previously submitted programme (including details of changes).
- Any future changes planned in respect of the programme (including details of proposed changes).
- A statistical return demonstrating the number of patients who have received an annual review.

Annual report

In addition, an annual report on the diabetes programme must be submitted to the FHSA. The following information will be requested:

- Confirmation that a *register of all diabetic patients in the practice* is in place and that it is regularly updated.
- Confirmation that the *clinical management programme* has proceeded as planned, that patients are being offered regular reviews and that call and recall systems are in place.
- Confirmation that all *practice nurses contributing to the programme have been appropriately trained,* giving names and details of courses in diabetes management attended.
- Confirmation that *attached staff* have contributed to the programmed as envisaged (with details).
- Confirmation that *records have been kept as planned* and if not, that details of changes have been made during the year.
- A *summary of any audit activities* undertaken in the programme area.
- *Additional information* regarding any activities in the programme area other than those originally submitted (with details).

- Completion of a *statistical return* regarding numbers, age, sex and whether insulin dependent or non-insulin dependent.
- Completion of *statistical return regarding number of annual reviews* (IDDM and NIDDM) carried out in hospital, shared care or by the practice alone.

Guidelines are supplied by FHSAs for the completion of the in-year monitoring return and annual report.

Reference

British Diabetic Association. Diabetes Services Advisory Committee (1993). *Recommendations for the Management of Diabetes in Primary Care: A revision of recommendations for diabetes health promotion clinics.*

16 Resources for the provision of diabetes care

Practical, useful and interesting books for people with diabetes

Title	Author	Publisher
Living with Non-insulin Dependent Diabetes*	John Day Susan Brenchley Suzanne Redmond	Medikos Ltd Mayfield House Harlequin Lane Crowborough East Sussex TN6 1HT
The Diabetes Handbook: Insulin Dependent Diabetes*	John Day	Thorsons Publishing Group 77-85 Fulham Palace Road London W6 8JB
Diabetes at your Fingertips: The Comprehensive Diabetes Reference Book for the 1990s	Peter Sonksen Charles Fox Sue Judd	Class Publishing Ltd 7 Melrose Terrace London W6 7RL
If Your Child is Diabetic*	Joanne Elliott	Sheldon Press Holy Trinity Church Marylebone Road London NW1 4DU
Teenage Diabetes*	Judith North	Thorsons Publishing Group (address above)
Diabetes and Pregnancy	Anna Knopfler	Little, Brown UK Ltd 165 Great Dover Street London SE1 4YA
Diabetes beyond 40	Rowan Hillson	Little, Brown UK Ltd (address above)

Titles marked * are available from the BDA.

| The Discovery of Insulin (out of print) | Michael Bliss | Macmillan Press Houndmills Basigstoke RG21 2XS |

Useful books for the primary care team

Title	Author	Publisher
Diabetes: Clinical Management	Tattersall R Gale E	Churchill Livingstone Burnt Mill Harlow Essex CM20 2JE
Diabetes in Practice	Connor H Boulton A	John Wiley and Sons Ltd Baffins Lane Chichester West Sussex PO19 1UD
Diabetes (in General Practice)	Waine C	Royal College of General Practitioners 14 Princess Gate London SW7 1PU
A Guide to the Provision of Health Care Services	Hill R D	Chapman and Hall 2-6 Boundary Row London SE1 8HN
Diabetes Care: A Problem Solving Approach (out of print)	Daly H Clarke P Field J	Heineman Medical Reed Distribution Services Rushden Northants NN10 9RZ
Exeter Diabetic Protocol, Third Edition 1993	Department of General Practice	University of Exeter Press Reed Hall Streatham Drive Exeter EX4 4QR
Diabetes and Primary Eye Care	Areffio A Hill R D Leigh O	Blackwell Scientific Publications Ltd Osney Mead Oxford OX2 0EL
A Colour Atlas of Ophthalmological Diagnosis Second Edition	Bedford M A	Mosby-Year Book Europe Ltd Brook House 2-16 Torrington Place London WC1 7LT

Journal of the Royal College of Physicians, Joint RCP/BDA recommendations for the management of NIDDM. In Press.

From the British Diabetic Association

Available from:
British Diabetic Association
10 Queen Anne Street
London W1M 0BD
Tel: 071 323-1531

Recommendations for the Management of Diabetes in Primary Care.
Diabetes Services Advisory Committee – March 1993

Diabetes Care – What you should expect – 1993

Minimal Educational Requirements for the Care of Diabetes in
the UK – 1987

Dietary Recommendations for People with Diabetes: An Update for the 1990s – 1993

General Practitioner Information Pack

The Diabetes Database. Information Department (for bibliographies, reports, articles)

For Posters, Leaflets, Books and Videos:
Catalogue and order form from BDA (available free).

Education in Diabetes – Courses and Conferences (send S A E with request)

'The Education Resources List' (in General Practitioner Information Pack) – lists educational materials available from Pharmaceutical/Equipment Companies

Balance – For People with Diabetes (free to members of the BDA)

Balance for Beginners – Insulin Dependent Diabetes (free)

Balance for Beginners – Non-insulin Dependent Diabetes (free)

Identification cards for IDDM and NIDDM

16

Journals

Diabetes Care, 4 issues per year available from:
Colwood House Medical Publications (UK) Ltd
Kirtons Farm　Pingewood
Reading　Berkshire RG3 3UN

Diabetes in General Practice, 4 issues per year available from:
Media Medica Publications Ltd
1 The Chambers　Chapel Street　Chichester　West Sussex PO19 1DL

Diabetic Medicine, 10 issues per year available from:
John Wiley and Sons Ltd
Baffins Lane　Chichester　West Sussex PO19 1UD

Diabetic Nursing, 3 issues per year (free) available from:
Media Medica Publications Ltd
1 The Chambers　Chapel Street　Chichester　West Sussex PO19 1DL

Diabetes Update, 2 issues per year (free) available from British Diabetic Association.

Practical Diabetes, 6 issues per year available from:
Media Medica Publications Ltd (Address above)

Companies

Providing equipment, booklets, leaflets, posters, videos, identification cards, monitoring diaries, GP information training, clinic packs, etc (local representatives will have specific details of what is available).

Bayer Diagnostics UK Limited (Ames Division)
Evans House, Hamilton Close　Basingstoke　Hampshire RG21 2YE
Tel: 0256 29181

Becton Dickinson UK Ltd
Between Towns Road　Cowley　Oxford OX4 3LY
Tel: 0865 748844

Boehringer Mannheim UK (BM)
Rapid Diagnostics Division　Bell Lane
Lewes　East Sussex BN7 1LG
Tel: 0273 480444

CP Pharmaceuticals (Fisons plc)
Coleorton Hall　Coleorton　Leicestershire LE6 4GP
Tel: 0509 634000

Farmitalia Carlo Erba Ltd
Italia House 23 Grosvenor Road St Albans Hertforshire AL1 3AW
Tel: 0727 40041

Hypoguard UK Ltd
Dock Lane Melton Woodridge Suffolk IP12 1PE
Tel: 0394 387333/4

Lilly Diabetes Care Division
Dextra Court Chapel Hill Basingstoke Hampshire
Tel: 0256 473241

Lipha Pharmaceuticals Ltd
Harrier House High Street Yiewsley West Drayton Middlesex UB7 7QG
Tel: 0895 449331

Medic-Alert Foundation
17 Bridge Wharf 156 Caledonian Road London N1 9UU
Tel: 071 833 3034

MediSense Britain Ltd
PO Box 20159 Coleshill Birmingham B46 1HZ
Tel: 0675 467044

Novo Nordisk Pharmaceuticals Ltd
Novo Nordisk House Broadfield Park Brighton Road Pease Pottage Crawley
West Sussex RH11 9RT
Tel: 0293 613555

16

Owen Mumford Ltd
Brook Hill Woodstock Oxford OX7 1TU
Tel: 0993 812021

Servier Laboratories Ltd
Metabolic Division Fulmer Hall Windmill Road Fulmer Slough
Buckinghamshire SL3 6HH
Tel: 0753 662744

SOS/Talisman
Golden Key Co Ltd 1 Hare Street Sheerness Kent ME12 1AH
Tel: 0795 663403

3M Heath Care Ltd
3M House Morley Street Loughborough Leicestershire LE11 0BR
Tel: 0509 611611

Other useful addresses

The English National Board for Nursing, Midwifery and Health Visiting
Victory House 170 Tottenham Court Road London W1P 9LS
Tel: 071 388 3131

The Manchester Diabetes Centre (Mrs Helen Siddons)
130 Hathersage Road Manchester M13 0HZ
Tel: 061 276 6700 Ext 6710

The Royal National Institute for the Blind
224 Great Portland Street London W1N 6AA
Tel: 071 388 1266

Life insurance and pensions

Brokers for BDA:
SBJ and Associates Ltd
National Westminster Bank Chambers
51 The Grove Gravesend Kent DA12 1DP
Tel: 0474 331166

Devitt Insurance Services Ltd
Central House 32-66 High Street London E15 2PP
Tel: 081 5190202

Part 3 About diabetes

17 Diabetes mellitus: a history of the condition

'Diabetes is a wonderful affection, not very frequent among men, being a melting down of the flesh and limbs into urine . . . life is short, disgusting and painful, thirst unquenchable, death inevitable'.

Aretaeus, the Cappadocian (2 AD)

Classification and types

Diabetes mellitus is a complex, metabolic disease characterised by high blood glucose concentrations. It is associated with impaired insulin production and/or action, resulting in the body's inability to utilise nutrients properly. It is believed that various genetic and environmental or lifestyle factors influence the cause and prognosis of the condition. Important differences in the frequency of diabetes and its complications have been reported between countries, ethnic and cultural groups.

The major clinical classes of glucose intolerance include insulin dependent diabetes mellitus (IDDM or Type I), non-insulin dependent diabetes mellitus (NIDDM or Type II), malnutrition related diabetes mellitus (MRDM), impaired glucose tolerance (IGT) and gestational diabetes (GDM). Terms and definitions used to describe and diagnose diabetes were unified and adopted in 1979-1980, updated in 1985 and reflected in the tenth revision of the International Statistical Classification of Diseases and related problems.

History

Diabetes has been known and recognised for many thousands of years as a disease characterised by weakness, thirst and frequency of micturition. Aretaeus, a contemporary of Galen, noted that the Greek word for a siphon had been given to diabetes because 'the fluid does not remain in the body, but uses the body as a ladder, whereby to leave it!'

Early treatments are described in the Ebers Papyrus written around 1500 BC, found in a grave in Thebes in Egypt in 1862. The treatment, 'to drive away the passing of too much urine. . . described a medicine including a mixture of bones, wheat grains, fresh fruits, green lead, earth and water. These ingredients the user should 'let stand moist, strain it, take it for 4 days'.

In modern times, the sweet taste of urine passed by people with this disease was noted by Willis in the late 17th century and Matthew Dobson of Liverpool demonstrated that the sweet taste was due to sugar. The Latin word for honey/sweet 'mellitus' was added to distinguish the disease from diabetes insipidus, a pituitary disorder, in which a large volume of sugar free urine is passed.

In 1815 the French chemist, Chevraul, showed that the sugar in diabetic urine was glucose. The association between diabetes and the pancreas was not recognised until much later. Paul Langerhans described the pancreatic islet cells in the mid-19th century and in 1889 Mering and Minkowski produced fatal diabetes by removing the pancreas in animals.

The real breakthrough came in 1921-22, when in Toronto Frederick Banting and Charles Best discovered insulin.

'Those who watched the first starved, sometimes comatose diabetics receive insulin and return to life saw one of the genuine miracles of modern medicine. They were present at the closest approach to the resurrection of the body that our secular society can achieve and at the discovery of what has become the elixir of life for millions of human beings around the world.'

So wrote Michael Bliss, the Canadian historian, in his definitive work on the discovery of insulin. Further research however revealed the complex physiology involved in the aetiology of the disease and in the development of complications. It was recognised that there were a number of different forms of diabetes. The discovery of insulin marked the therapeutic period. It confirmed the concept of a deficiency of insulin action as the basic abnormality in diabetes and gave rise to the differentiation between insulin dependent diabetes mellitus (IDDM) and non-insulin dependent diabetes mellitus (NIDDM).

Pharmaceutical research and development relating to IDDM has concentrated on developing 'purer' and more effective forms of insulin and new methods of delivery by 'pens' and 'pumps', although the latter have failed to live up to their early promise. Genetically engineered human insulin was introduced in the mid-1980s and in many countries it is a substitute for insulin of animal origin.

Oral hypoglycaemic agents were first introduced in Germany in 1955 and have been extensively developed. There are two main groups, the sulphonylureas and the biguanides. The sulphonylureas act mainly by stimulating the release of insulin from the beta cells in the pancreas. The action of the biguanide group is less clear but is believed to increase the peripheral uptake of glucose.

Diet is the 'cornerstone' of treatment. An interesting observation on the effect of food on the incidence and progression of diabetes was made by the French physician Bouchardat in 1875, during the Prussian siege of Paris. The siege was prolonged and as food supplies ran out, forcing the population to eat cats and dogs, he noticed the absence of new cases in his practice and an improvement in the condition of those already diagnosed. Similar observations were made in the two world wars when national death rates for diabetes noticeably fell.

Dietary recommendations have changed from a restricted carbohydrate intake to a regime low in fat and high in unrefined carbohydrates and dietary fibre. For the overweight, reduction in energy intake remains the most important aim. Carbohydrate should make up about 50-55% of the energy intake, preferably from foods naturally high in dietary fibre. Up to 25 g of added sucrose per day may be allowed provided it is part of a diet low in fat and high in fibre.

Dietary advice in the treatment of diabetes is not only aimed at the control of blood glucose but also at the prevention of cardiovascular disease. In general it is the same advice as that offered to the general population.

The discovery of insulin by Banting and Best highlighted and accelerated the quest for understanding of the condition. As more has become known, the search for the causes of diabetes has moved towards further study of the immune system, the role of infection and the genetic implications already identified.

References

Besser, G M; Bodansky, H J; Cudworth A G (1988). *Clinical Diabetes – An Illustrated Text.* Gower Medical Publishing.

Bliss, M (1983). *The Discovery of Insulin.* Macmillan Press.

British Diabetic Association Report (1992). *Dietary Recommendations for people with diabetes.* Diabetic Medicine 9:189-202.

Day, J L (1986). *The Diabetes Handbook – Non-Insulin Dependent Diabetes.* Thorsons Publishing Group.

Laing, W; Williams, R (1989). *Diabetes: a Model for Health Care Management.* Office of Health Economics.

18 Insulin dependent diabetes (IDDM)

Formerly termed acute diabetes or juvenile onset diabetes, this type commonly occurs in childhood, adolescence and on into adult life. Symptoms of profound weight loss, excessive thirst, polyuria, lethargy and occasionally abdominal pain require immediate treatment with insulin. Should treatment not be available, ketoacidosis, coma and death are inevitable. The onset is sudden (days or weeks).

Diagnosis

Diagnosis is usually straightforward, based on the presenting symptoms and raised blood glucose levels (greater than 11.1 mmol/l venous plasma or greater than 12.2 mmol/l capillary plasma). Following diagnosis, insulin therapy is commenced together with appropriate family support and education about living with diabetes in all its aspects. Discussion about modification of food intake and activity in relation to the person's life are staged alongside the stabilisation process. A careful multi-disciplinary approach with empathy and consistent, correct advice are vital in fostering a healthy 'life with insulin' and in the reduction of acute and long term complications.

Two acute complications (hypoglycaemia and hyperglycaemia) occur in relation to insulin therapy and are associated with the extremes of blood glucose levels.

Hypoglycaemia

Hypoglycaemia (blood glucose levels below 4 mmol/l) may occur with little warning, due to too much insulin, insufficient food, delayed meals, alcohol, extra activity or stress.

Hyperglycaemia

Hyperglycaemia (blood glucose levels above 13 mmol/l; progressing to higher levels) is the second acute complication of insulin therapy. Vomiting, dehydration and ketosis will develop into severe fluid depletion, disordered blood chemistry and electrolyte imbalance which, if uncorrected, may be irreversible and death will follow. This situation occurs during illness or may occur where the psychological state is severely affected resulting in the person using insulin as a tool of manipulation.

Improved support services and the development of technology allowing people with diabetes the opportunity to check their own blood glucose levels has, over many years, now greatly improved their confidence in the self-management of their insulin therapy and in the prevention of occasions of 'acute complications'. This self-regulation of blood glucose is particularly important during pregnancy, where strict blood glucose control is vital even before conception. Pre-pregnancy counselling and blood glucose levels between 4 mmol/l and 7 mmol/l are essential to avoid foetal abnormality or death. Thirty years ago, about one quarter of diabetic pregnancies ended in foetal death. Now almost all are successful. This improvement is due to major developments in obstetric, diabetic and paediatric care. Major congenital abnormalities however still occur more frequently than in non-diabetic pregnancies.

The causes of insulin dependent diabetes

Factors involved in the causation of insulin dependent diabetes are complex. Genetic factors are not only involved but also environmental factors, demonstrated by changes in islet cells and destruction of beta cells, either directly or by triggering an auto-immune response. Possible environmental agents suggested are infective conditions (perhaps occurring some years before) as well as physical, chemical and psychological factors.

The prevalence of IDDM varies considerably in different countries, based on estimates, varying levels of ascertainment and population age structure. Prevalence appears to be higher further from the Equator, in particular in Scandinavia, and lower than average in Japan.

Seasonal variations in incidence are also of interest as they are consistent and occur all over the world. Higher incidence rates are reported during the autumn and winter months than over the spring and summer periods. Seasonal variations are thought to be associated with the presence of infective agents such as viruses. These may trigger the onset of the disease in susceptible people, in particular young people where incidence is age related and peaks around the ages of 5 and 12 years coinciding with changes of school environments and the onset of puberty.

In summary

1. The prevalence of IDDM is approximately one tenth that of NIDDM in western communities.

2. Clinical onset occurs during childhood particularly around the time of puberty.

3. The condition also appears in early and later adulthood.

4. There is a higher incidence in autumn and winter and an increasing gradient in incidence from southern to northern latitudes.

References

Bramer, G R (1988). *International statistical classification of disease and health related problems – Tenth Revision.* World Health Statistics Quarterly 41:32-36.

Laing, W; Williams, R (1989). *Diabetes: a Model for Health Care Management.* Office of Health Economics.

Pyke, D A and Nelson, P E (1976). *Diabetes mellitus in identical twins.* In: The Genetics of Diabetes Mellitus. Edited by Crevtzfeldt, W; Kobbenking, J and Neel, J V 194-202. Springer Verlag, Berlin.

Rewers, M et al (1988). *Trends in the prevalence and incidence of diabetes. Insulin dependent diabetes in childhood.* World Health Statistics Quarterly 41:179-189.

Watkins, P J (1988). *ABC of Diabetes.* British Medical Journal.

WHO Technical Report Series No 727 (1985). *Diabetes mellitus.* Report of a WHO Study Group, Geneva WHO.

19 Non-insulin dependent diabetes mellitus (NIDDM)

NIDDM, the most common form of diabetes, increases in prevalence from 30-35 years of age. By 70 years of age, prevalence is usually three to four times higher than the overall prevalence in adults (2%-5% in European and North American Communities). *Undiagnosed,* almost exclusively, NIDDM has been reported in nearly equal proportions to diagnosed diabetes in many societies.

In developing countries, NIDDM is rare in the traditional setting but has become very common, exceeding 1%, in adults in many urbanised communities. Several ethnic groups have a greater genetic predisposition to NIDDM than do Caucasians. In the absence of effective interventions, the prevalence of NIDDM in all populations is likely to rise, due to ageing, a reduction in infectious disease mortality and increases in the prevalence of obesity, lack of regular physical exercise and inappropriate diet.

Efforts to prevent obesity through diet alone have been generally unsuccessful. Physical activity however appears to have an important role in the prevention of NIDDM through its association with reduced body weight and through independent effects on insulin resistance and glucose tolerance. Further research is needed to assess the magnitude of the benefits of exercise and to determine the most effective exercise programmes for reducing the incidence of NIDDM. To date, research has failed to demonstrate an association between NIDDM and specific genetic markers even though it is a familial disease.

Both sexes are affected in non-insulin dependent diabetes, although in some communities a male preponderance is shown, for example in India and in Asian Indians in the United Kingdom. In others the majority with the disease are female. In populations where NIDDM is common it may be encountered in adolescence and among young adults. This form of diabetes, which has a familial distribution compatible with a dominant mode of inheritance, is sometimes referred to as mature onset diabetes of the young (MODY).

Diagnosis

The diagnosis of non-insulin dependent diabetes is less clear cut than that of IDDM (see Fig 19.1). Hitherto, the condition has been called 'mild' diabetes of maturity onset; it is rare below the age of 35 years (when it is likely to be termed MODY). The onset is insidious and may only be revealed at routine screening. Symptoms of lethargy, thirst and polyuria are the most common but may proceed unnoticed until an episode of stress or an infection precipitate the severity of symptoms, forcing the individual to seek help. The diagnosis will be established by raised blood glucose levels (venous blood greater than 8 mmol/l fasting or random levels of greater than 11 mmol/l).

Should blood glucose levels be raised but less than these values, a glucose tolerance test should be performed by the patient taking 75 g of glucose under specified conditions and, following a measurement of a fasting blood glucose level, sequential blood glucose levels are then tested. The results are interpreted according to WHO criteria to confirm the presence or absence of diabetes or the existence of impaired glucose tolerance.

Treatment

Treatment for people with non-insulin dependent diabetes is aimed at the alleviation of symptoms, the reduction of blood glucose levels and where possible, the prevention of complications. Should the patient be overweight the first line of treatment consists of dietary modification and education to reduce weight. If successful, this may lead to a reduction in blood glucose levels and symptomatic relief.

Should this line of treatment be unsuccessful, oral hypoglycaemic agents may be required. Should these fail to achieve the desired result, insulin therapy may be required. The normal weight or underweight person unable to obtain symptom relief and/or reduction in blood glucose levels with dietary modification and hypoglycaemic agents will usually require insulin sooner rather than later.

Extreme caution is required in treatment with oral hypoglycaemic agents (and insulin therapy) in the elderly, in order to avoid the complication of hypoglycaemia. People with non-insulin dependent diabetes may require insulin in the short term in times of illness or during a surgical intervention. The complications of insulin treatment in NIDDM are those of hypoglycaemia and weight gain. The problem of hypoglycaemia often deters the instigation of this therapy. A short term 'trial' of insulin may provide the answer as to the best course of treatment.

Combined regimes of oral hypoglycaemic agents (sulphonylureas) and insulin have been used in some centres but to little advantage. The livelihood of people with diabetes also must be considered. People holding particular types of driving licences such as Large Goods Vehicle (LGV) and Public Service Vehicle (PSV) will lose these should insulin therapy be instituted. A most difficult problem to be solved occurs when insulin is used in the treatment of symptomless people with NIDDM, where weight gain progresses with no improvement in blood glucose levels.

Fig 19.1 Differences between insulin dependent diabetes (IDDM) and non-insulin dependent diabetes.

	IDDM	NIDDM
Proportions %	25%	75%
Usual age of onset	Under 30 years	Over 30 years
Speed of onset	Rapid	Gradual
Likelihood of ketosis	High	Low
Complications at presentation	No	Yes, frequently
Treatment	Diet and insulin	Diet alone, diet and tablets, or diet and insulin
Likelihood of hypoglycaemia	More	Less but dangerous in the elderly
Precipitated by obesity	No	Yes
Majority of care provision	Hospital	General Practitioner

In summary

1. Non-insulin dependent diabetes is common, affecting 2%-5% of the population, rising with age.

2. The onset usually occurs after the age of 35 years.

3. NIDDM is not a 'mild condition'. It is associated with considerable morbidity and mortality.

4. Weight gain and physical inactivity are important factors in the progress of the condition.

5. Treatment is complex, particularly in older people.

References

Besser, G M; Bodansky, H J; Cudworth, A G (1988) *Clinical Diabetes – An Illustrated Text.* Gower Medical Publishing, London.

British Diabetic Association (1988). *Diabetes in the United Kingdom.* British Diabetic Association, London.

Day, J L (1986) *The Diabetes Handbook – Non-Insulin Dependent Diabetes.* Thorsons Publishing Group, London.

European NIDDM Policy Group (1989). *A Desktop Guide for the Management of Non-Insulin Dependent Diabetes Mellitus* (NIDDM). Boehringer Mannheim GmbH, Mannheim FRG.

Harris, M I (1987). *Prevalence of diabetes and impaired glucose tolerance in US population aged 20-74 years.* Diabetes 36:523-34.

Manson, J E et al (1991). *Physical activity and incidence of non-insulin dependent diabetes in women.* Lancet 338:774-778.

O'Rahilly, S et al (1988). *Type II (non-insulin dependent diabetes mellitus) New genetics for old nightmares.* Diabetologia 31:407414.

Peacock, I; Tattersall, R B (1984). *The difficult choice of treatment for poorly controlled maturity onset diabetes: tablets or insulin?* British Medical Journal 288:1956-1959.

Rudermann, M; Apelian, A Z; Schneider, S M (1990). *Exercise in therapy and prevention of type II diabetes: implications for blacks.* Diabetes Care 13 (suppl 4):1163-68.

20 Other categories of diabetes

Impaired glucose tolerance

The US National Diabetes Data Group introduced the category of impaired glucose tolerance (IGT) in 1979 and this was later endorsed by the WHO Expert Committee Report No 646 in 1980.

Previously, the term 'borderline' diabetes had been used to distinguish between people whose glucose tolerance was 'impaired' in relation to the non-diabetic population but who were not frankly diabetic. The IGT category removed the label of 'diabetes' since this level of glucose intolerance is not associated with the development of microvascular complications.

Impaired glucose tolerance is however, associated with increased risk of death from ischaemic heart disease. A proportion of people with IGT progress to diabetes within a few years. Estimates range from 1% to 5% depending on age and subsequent duration of follow up.

Gestational diabetes mellitus

Gestational diabetes is defined as carbohydrate intolerance of variable severity with onset or first recognition during the present pregnancy. The definition applies, whether insulin is used for treatment, or the condition persists after pregnancy but does not exclude the possibility that the glucose intolerance may have ante-dated the pregnancy (American Diabetes Association 1991). This abnormal glucose intolerance is generally indicated by a fasting venous blood glucose concentration of 6 mmol/l or above. It is extremely unlikely that such a fasting level would occur in a non-diabetic woman. A fasting level of 6 mmol/l or above is associated with increased morbidity in the foetus.

Generally, gestational diabetes resolves post-partum. The condition includes those with a genetic or acquired susceptibility, in whom the metabolic changes of pregnancy induce a temporary diabetic state. People with a 'low level' of diabetes present before pregnancy, become symptomatic and are diagnosed at routine screening during antenatal care.

It is important that women at risk of developing gestational diabetes are identified, as the condition is associated with an increased incidence of perinatal morbidity and the development of diabetes by the mother in later life.

Antenatal care should include the following assessment
1. Previous gestational diabetes or impaired glucose tolerance.
2. Family history of diabetes.
3. Maternal obesity (>120% ideal body weight).
4. Previous delivery of a large baby.
5. Previous unexplained still birth.
6. Certain ethnic groups (Indo-Pakistani women in central London have an 8.6% incidence of an abnormal glucose tolerance test).
7. Women over 25 years of age.
8. Previous obstetric and/or perinatal complications.
9. Recurrent urinary tract infections or candidiasis.

Once the history is known, those 'at risk' are identified for testing. Owing to the low renal threshold that exists in pregnancy, urine testing is of little value. Overt diabetes is missed and only a few of those with impaired glucose tolerance are identified. The best compromise is a 75 g oral dose of glucose followed one hour later by a plasma glucose measurement. A full oral glucose tolerance test is impractical for screening the antenatal population although it is the only definitive test for the diagnosis of gestational diabetes.

The management of gestational diabetes involves intensive team work between obstetric and diabetes carers and involves support for the woman throughout pregnancy. Tight blood glucose control with dietary modification and/or insulin therapy is required, similar to a pregnant woman with established diabetes, to avoid antenatal complications and perinatal morbidity and mortality. Oral hypoglycaemic agents are not used in the treatment of gestational diabetes or diabetes, in pregnancy. Particular support is required for women with gestational diabetes when they are first diagnosed in order that treatment can be commenced quickly and blood glucose levels lowered as soon as possible. Obstetric management is similar to that provided for women with diabetes.

Following delivery, a full oral glucose tolerance test is performed 6 to 8 weeks post-partum. Advice is given regarding the maintenance of ideal body weight and that gestational diabetes may recur in subsequent pregnancies. Should the glucose tolerance test be abnormal, referral to a diabetes team for follow up is required and treatment, support and further education provided.

It is generally accepted that 40% of women with gestational diabetes will develop diabetes within 20 years. This is usually of the non-insulin dependent type. An awareness of this is of importance in the avoidance of long term complications of diabetes.

References

Beard, R W; Moet, J J (1982). *Is gestational diabetes a clinical entity?* Diabetologia 23:307-312.

Chahal, P (1988). *Diabetes and Pregnancy.* Butterworths, London.

Oakley, C E (1992). *Care of gestational diabetes.* Diabetes Care 1:6-8.

20

21 Other causes of diabetes – secondary diabetes

There are many disorders or syndromes associated with secondary diabetes. Relatively, however, they account for a small number of patients with the condition.

Hormonal causes of diabetes

Overt diabetes or glucose intolerance is often associated with Cushing's Syndrome. If the causative tumour is removed or the Cushing's Syndrome treated, the diabetes can be improved or even cured.

Approximately a third of patients with acromegaly develop diabetes which improves on treatment of the acromegalic condition. Phaeochromocytoma also produces glucose intolerance which may be intermittent.

Patients with tumours producing corticosteroids, acid ACTH, growth hormone, glucagon and catecholamines all induce insulin resistance.

Pancreatic disease

Severe disease of the pancreas or pancreatectomy causes diabetes which may require insulin therapy. As glucagon is absent following these pancreatic conditions, control of the diabetes is erratic and may require only small doses of insulin – or severe hypoglycaemia results. Acute pancreatitis, cystic fibrosis and chronic pancreatitis may cause diabetes.

Carcinoma of the pancreas

The appearance of diabetes and jaundice almost simultaneously, usually within a few weeks, suggests the diagnosis of this condition. When surgery is indicated, insulin therapy will almost always be required.

Haemochromatosis

A condition of defective iron metabolism results in the accumulation of iron in the tissues and over-absorption of iron which may result in the concentration of iron in the liver and pancreas 50–100 times normal levels. Other endocrine glands show heavy iron deposits. Patients with this condition are usually male, aged 40 to 60 years, with a ratio of 9 to 1 (males to females). Two-thirds of people with haemochromatosis have diabetes, usually requiring insulin.

Drug induced diabetes

Thiazides reduce glucose tolerance by impairing insulin secretion. Thiazide diuretics may have a significant hyperglycaemic effect in non-insulin dependent diabetes.

Corticosteroids impair glucose tolerance mainly by increasing glucose production and increasing insulin resistance. Diabetic control is worsened by corticosteroids soon after administration. These drugs may precipitate diabetes; they do not cause the condition unless large doses are used, as in transplant therapy, to counter rejection episodes. Diabetes is most likely to occur in people who have had impaired glucose tolerance or gestational diabetes. Thyroxine may impair glucose tolerance although not sufficiently to alter diabetic control. The combined oestrogen-progestogen contraceptive pill only mildly impairs glucose tolerance and does not effect diabetic control in insulin dependent diabetes.

Tumours of the islet cells

Glucagonoma is a rare tumour of the islet secreting A-cells, producing characteristic clinical features, skin rashes, anaemia, thrombo-embolic disease and diabetes. A very rare tumour is a somatostatinoma of the D-cells and is commonly associated with diabetes.

Insulinomae are tumours of the islet cells containing large amounts of insulin causing hypoglycaemia in people who do not have diabetes. Surgical removal of the tumour usually cures this condition.

Hereditary causes

There are around 50 genetic syndromes associated with clinical diabetes or impaired glucose tolerance. These, however, are rare. Examples of well documented genetic syndromes are:

DIDMOAD syndrome (diabetes insipidus, diabetes mellitus, optic atrophy and deafness) is recessively inherited and insulin dependent diabetes is associated with the development of diabetes insipidus, blindness from optic atrophy and gradual onset of high tone deafness.

Mature onset of diabetes in the young (MODY) is also known as Mason's syndrome and follows a pattern of dominant inheritance. Occurring in the young, the person affected remains non-insulin requiring for many years. Long term complications associated with this syndrome are less common. (The term Mason relates to the first family in whom the syndrome was recognised).

Other disorders associated with secondary diabetes are Addison's Disease (more common in people with insulin dependent diabetes than in the general population), hypopituitarism and thyroid disease.

Malnutrition related diabetes mellitus (MRDM)

A significant proportion of younger people (onset usually below 30 years of age) in tropical developing countries do not fall into either of the two main classes of diabetes (IDDM and NIDDM). These people have a particular set of symptoms and metabolic types to justify special categorisation. Malnutrition related diabetes may constitute 30%-60% of all cases of young onset diabetes in developing countries.

In summary

Secondary causes of diabetes

1. Hormonal

2. Pancreatic disease

3. Carcinoma of the pancreas

4. Haemochromatosis

5. Drug induced – especially steroids and thiazides

6. Tumours of the islet cells

7. Hereditary causes

8. Malnutrition related diabetes (seen in developing countries)

References

Bajaj, J S (Ed) (1984). *Malnutrition related diabetes.* In: Diabetes Mellitus in Developing Countries. Interprint Publishers. New Delhi.

Bajaj, J S and Subbaro, B (1988). *Malnutrition related diabetes mellitus.* In: World Book of Diabetes in Practice Vol 3:25. Elsevier Science Publishers BV (Biomedical Division).

Laing, W; Williams, R (1989). *Diabetes: a Model for Health Care Management.* Office of Health Economics.

Siddle, N C; Knight, M A (1991). *Managing the Menopause. A Practical Guide to HRT.* Medical Communications Services, Oxted RH8 0TF.

Watkins, P J; Drury, P L; Taylor, K W (1990). *Diabetes and its Management.* Blackwell Scientific Publications.

21

22 The complications of diabetes

Two important factors in the causation of complications of diabetes are:

• Hyperglycaemia
• The duration of diabetes.

The long term complications of insulin dependent diabetes, those of *nephropathy, retinopathy, autonomic and peripheral neuropathy* are rarely seen before 5 to 7 years duration of the condition. Most commonly they do not occur before 10 to 20 years. In non-insulin dependent diabetes, however, complications may be present at diagnosis, the condition having been unrecognised for several years prior to presentation. As duration of diabetes lengthens, complications may progress, although after 30 years' duration, the annual incidence decreases. Some people with diabetes of 30 to 60 years duration are free from the long term complications of the condition.

Other factors in the development of complications are vascular changes which are affected by metabolic dysfunction. Genetic markers of susceptibility have not been identified. The eyes, the kidneys and the peripheral nerves are organs most affected by diabetes. These organs may be affected to a different extent, one being severely affected while another is not damaged at all. The 'hallmark' of long standing diabetes is the thickening of basement membrane which can be observed in the kidney, retina, nerves, skin, muscle and adipose tissue. Biochemical dysfunction is also identified as a possible problem in relation to the glycosylation of proteins and pathways of sorbitol. Associations exist between the major complications of diabetes, with patterns of association more marked in insulin dependent diabetes (such as retinopathy, nephropathy and neuropathy in the same person) than in the non-insulin dependent diabetes type.

In summary

Major complications of diabetes

Specific

1. Renal disease   Diabetic nephropathy

2. Eye disease   Background retinopathy

                          Proliferative retinopathy

3. Neuropathy   Autonomic neuropathy

                          Peripheral neuropathy

                          Cranial nerve palsies

                          Peripheral mononeuropathy

Increased frequency of other diseases

1. Cardiac problems   Coronary heart disease

2. Eyes   Cataracts

Some specific complications

Renal disease – diabetic nephropathy

Diabetic nephropathy is recognised as a major cause of morbidity and mortality in people with insulin dependent diabetes affecting some 40% of patients developing the disease before the age of 31 years. Reliable information regarding nephropathy in people with non-insulin dependent diabetes is less available, as precise identification of the onset of this condition is difficult to ascertain. However, the relative risk of death from renal failure in this group is thought to be lower in older patients. The problem is still a major one in terms of prevalence as 75% – 90% of people with diabetes are non-insulin dependent. It is reported that between 32% – 90% of this large group enter treatment programmes for end stage renal disease.

Next to glomerulonephritis, diabetes is ranked as the commonest cause for patients requiring renal dialysis and transplantation. A specific type of renal lesion occurs in the glomerular capillaries known as diabetic glomerulosclerosis.

Diabetic renal failure and its progression can be described in four stages.

Stage 1 – At initial diagnosis of insulin dependent diabetes, a 24 hour urine collection will show an elevated glomerular filtration rate as high as 160 ml/min (normal level – 120 ml/min). This is known as supra-filtration. This abnormality is reversible with insulin treatment over a period of weeks or months. However, a normal glomerular filtration rate is usually never achieved. The patient is said to continually hyperfiltrate leading in the long term to structural damage in the glomerulus.

Stage 2 – Taking on average 10 to 15 years to reach this stage, damaged glomeruli allow the passage of clinically undetectable amounts of protein to be filtered into the urine. This is termed *microalbuminuria*. The importance of lower concentrations of albumin excretion has been recognised in recent years. Microalbuminuria has been applied to an albumin excretion rate of 30-300 mg/day. This level of increased albumin excretion would not be identified on standard dipstick testing for proteinuria (eg with Albustix, Unstix or Multistix) but has been shown in patients with IDDM to be highly predictive of progression to overt nephropathy and renal failure in people with insulin dependent diabetes. In non-insulin dependent diabetes, studies have suggested a prevalence of microalbuminuria of 12%-16%. The prevalence of this condition is higher in certain ethnic groups. It is more common in people from the Indian sub-continent than in Caucasians in the United Kingdom.

Microalbuminuria can now be detected using stick or tablet tests (eg from Boehringer Mannheim or Nycomed (UK) Ltd and once it is noted, it indicates incipient diabetic renal failure, progressing to clinical diabetic nephropathy, possibly requiring dialysis in the future.

Stage 3 – Overt diabetic renal failure is present at this stage. Proteinuria can be detected by Albustix testing. Severe proteinuria presents as nephrotic syndrome. At this stage, the glomerular filtration rate starts to decline with *rising serum urea and creatinine* levels, indicating diabetic renal failure.

Stage 4 – Finally, the glomerular filtration rate is no longer able to maintain haemostasis, resulting in end stage renal failure, requiring dialysis or renal transplantation.

Delaying the progression of diabetic nephropathy
There are three main elements of treatment involved in the delay of the progression of diabetic nephropathy.

Detection and control of raised blood pressure
Detection and control of raised blood pressure by aggressive hypertensive treatment postpones renal insufficiency in diabetic nephropathy.

Glycaemic control
If this is achieved in the early stages of the condition, albumin excretion may be reduced.

Protein restriction in the diet (in IDDM)
Has been found to have a beneficial effect on microalbuminuria, independent of changes in glucose concentrations and arterial blood pressure.

Once renal failure is established haemodialysis, continuous ambulatory peritoneal dialysis (CAPD) or renal transplantation are the only options available for the continuation of life.

Tests for microalbuminuria

Stick test	*Tablet test*
Boehringer Mannheim UK (BM)	Nycomed (UK) Limited
Bell Lane	2111 Coventry Road
Lewes	Birmingham
East Sussex	B26 3EA
BN7 1LG	Tel: 021 742 2444
Tel: 0273 480444	

In summary

Diabetic nephropathy

1. Affects 40% of people with IDDM diagnosed before the age of 31 years.

2. Affects 32%-90% of people with NIDDM although figures less accurate as duration of NIDDM may not be known.

3. There are four stages of diabetic renal disease.

4. Microalbuminuria may be detected at Stage 2 following 10-15 years of diabetes.

5. Microalbuminuria can be detected using simple tests.

6. Raised serum urea and creatinine levels (Stage 3) indicate renal failure.

7. Delaying the progression of diabetic nephropathy involves three elements of treatment:

a) Detection and control of raised blood pressure

b) Glycaemic control

c) In IDDM – dietary protein restriction *may* be of benefit

8. Established renal failure will require the following treatment options:

a) Haemodialysis

b) CAPD

c) Renal transplantation

Eye disease – diabetic retinopathy

Diabetic retinopathy encompasses the retino-vascular complications of diabetes. It is one of the major causes of blindness in developed countries. 2% of the diabetic population have been estimated to be blind from diabetic retinopathy. In people under the age of 65 years, it is the most common cause of blindness, accounting for 19.7% of all new registrations in the 16 to 64 age group.

The incidence of diabetic retinopathy is closely related to the duration of diabetes and its progression is variable from slow to rapid onset. The frequency of diabetic retinopathy is increasing with the greater longevity of the diabetic population. It is estimated that after 10 years of diabetic life, 20% will have diabetic retinopathy and after 20 years, 80% of the diabetic population will be affected. L'Esperance estimated that 60% of people with diabetes with a duration of the disease for more than 15 years will have some form of retinopathy with females more commonly affected.

Diabetic retinopathy is rare in children, although it may occur, usually following the onset of puberty. This is thought to be due to growth increase, hormonal changes and poor glycaemic control.

Background retinopathy
Microaneurysms, haemorrhages and yellow white patches in rings (hard exudates) are characteristic and are harmless unless they occur on the macula (area

of vision). Should the macula be oedematous, blindness may occur if this condition is not treated.

Proliferative retinopathy
Formation of 'new vessels' (pre-proliferative retinopathy) due to retinal ischaemia is a dangerous sign and may proceed to *proliferative retinopathy* and haemorrhage, causing retinal detachment and other severe ocular disorders leading to visual impairment and blindness.

Screening
For visual impairment and blindness to be averted, people with diabetes should be identified and screened (annually). Visual acuity should be checked at regular intervals, as deteriorating vision may indicate the presence of sight threatening retinopathy, although normal visual acuity may occur even though retinopathy is present. Following this test, examination of the fundi through dilated pupils should be carried out, to determine the presence or progress of retinopathy.

There is good evidence that improved patient education and regular screening programmes combined with early detection of retinal changes and photocoagulation therapy, have major effects on reducing visual impairment and blindness in diabetes mellitus.

In summary

Diabetic retinopathy

1. Diabetic retinopathy is one of the major causes of blindness in developed countries.

2. It accounts for nearly 20% of blindness in the 16-64 age group.

3. The incidence of retinopathy is related to the duration of diabetes.

4. The onset of retinopathy may be rapid or slow.

5. There are three main categories of diabetic retinopathy:

a) Background retinopathy

b) Pre-proliferative retinopathy

c) Proliferative retinopathy

6. People with diabetes should be identified and their eyes screened annually.

7. A screening programme should include testing for visual acuity and examination of the fundi through dilated pupils.

8. Patient education, regular screening, early detection of retinal change and photocoagulation therapy reduce visual impairment and blindness.

Diabetic neuropathy

Autonomic neuropathy

It is estimated that 20%-40% of all people with diabetes have some abnormality of autonomic function. Insidious in onset, its presence may be undetected until late in its natural history. Dysfunction may be present in the cardiovascular system (causing postural hypotension), the alimentary tract (causing uncontrollable diarrhoea), the respiratory control system and in thermo-regulation. Genito-urinary disturbances are also distressing; one of the major problems being that of impotence. It has been reported that 50% of men with diabetes eventually become impotent. Few men attending diabetic clinics seek help and fewer are treated, although several effective treatments are now available.

Peripheral neuropathy

About 20% of people with diabetes have neuropathy affecting peripheral nerves, mainly those of the feet and legs. More hospital beds in Britain are occupied by diabetic patients with lower limb and foot problems than with all the other complications of diabetes combined. The two main features are neuropathy and ischaemia, often present together. Identification of those at risk of foot ulceration and preventative education are the most important aspects of the care of the neuropathic foot in the person with diabetes and in the prevention of prolonged hospital admission and amputation.

In summary

Diabetic neuropathy

1. Autonomic neuropathy affects 20%-40% of all people with diabetes.

2. Autonomic neuropathy may affect many body systems.

3. Autonomic neuropathy causes impotence in 50% of men with diabetes. Treatment for this condition is available.

4. Peripheral neuropathy affects 20% of people with diabetes.

5. Lower limb and foot problems due to peripheral neuropathy and ischaemia are common causing prolonged hospital admission and amputation.

6. Identification of those at risk of foot ulceration and education are important preventative measures.

Increased frequency of other diseases

Cardiac disease and diabetes mellitus

Heart disease is a common cause of morbidity and mortality in people with diabetes. The Framingham study demonstrated that people with diabetes have increased morbidity and mortality from all cardiovascular causes which persist when the risk factors of hyperlipidaemia, hypertension and obesity are taken into account. The increased incidence of coronary artery disease in male and female diabetic patients was 60% in males and 100% in females respectively, compared with values for non-diabetic individuals.

Epidemiological studies have demonstrated that even mild impairment of glucose tolerance is associated with an increase in atherosclerosis. This may imply that hyperglycaemia is an important factor, although it is possible that other factors, as yet unidentified, are involved. Hypertension is approximately twice as common in diabetic patients as in age matched people without diabetes. It is more frequent in insulin dependent diabetes than in non-insulin dependent diabetes. Obesity and the presence of renal disease are associated with hypertension in diabetes, however, it has been shown that these links extend further. Epidemiologically, there is an association between blood glucose levels (after a standard load) and both systolic and diastolic blood pressure, independent of body weight.

Cataracts and diabetes mellitus

The association between cataracts and diabetes is well known. Cataracts may indicate the presence of diabetes and are more common in people with diabetes. It has also been shown that there is a significant association between the prevalence of cataract and age as well as duration of diabetes. This is important, as progression of this condition leading to severe visual impairment has profound implications on living with diabetes, quality of life and health care costs.

In summary

Cardiac disease and diabetes mellitus

1. Diabetes increases (by two or three times) the risk of cardiac disease – a common cause of morbidity and mortality.

2. Hyperglycaemia is an important factor.

3. Other important factors are thought to be involved, but not yet identified.

4. Hypertension is more frequent in IDDM than in NIDDM.

References

Anderson, A R; Christiansen, J S; Anderson A K et al (1983). *Diabetic Nephropathy in Type I (insulin dependent) Diabetes, An Epidemiological Study.* Diabetologia 25:496-501.

Caird, F I; Pirie, A and Ramsell, T G (1969). In: *Diabetes and the Eye.* Blackwell Scientific Publications.

Carroll, R (1992). *Kidney damage in diabetes.* Nursing Vol 5; No 6:17-20.

Deckert, T; Pulsen, J E; Larsen, M (1978). *Prognosis of diabetes with diabetes before the age of 31.* Diabetologia 14:363-70.

Diabetic Retinopathy Study Research Group (1981). *Photocoagulation treatment of proliferative diabetic retinopathy: clinical application of diabetic retinopathy study (DRS) findings.* DRS Report No 8. Ophthalmol 88:583-600.

Edmonds, M E (1985). *The neuropathic ulcer.* Practical Diabetes Vol 2; No 1:46-47

Elkeles, R S; Wolfe, J H N (1991). *The diabetic foot.* British Medical Journal 303:1053-1055.

Geiss, L S; Herman, W H; Teutsch, S M (1985). *Diabetes and renal mortality in the United States.* American Journal of Public Health 75:1325-6.

Hale, P J (1984). *Why do diabetic patients suffer from coronary artery disease?* Practical Diabetes Vol 1; No 2:22-35.

HMSO (1988). *Causes of blindness and partial sight amongst adults.* HMSO, London.

Joint Working Party on Diabetic Renal Failure of the British Diabetic Association, The Renal Association and The Research Unit of The Royal College of Physicians (1988). *Renal failure in the UK: deficient provision of care in 1985.* Diabetic Medicine 5:79-84.

Kannel, W B; McGee, D C (1979). *Diabetes and cardiovascular disease: The Framingham Study.* Journal of the American Medical Association 241:2035-8.

Klein, B E; Klein, R and Moss, S E (1985). *Prevalence of cataracts in a population based study of persons with diabetes mellitus.* Ophthalmology 92:1191-6.

Kohner, E M (1978). *The evolution and natural history of diabetic retinopathy.* Int Ophthalmol Clin 18:1-16.

McCulloch, D K; Young, R J; Prescott, I W et al (1984). *The natural history of impotence in diabetic men.* Diabetologia 26:437-40.

Mogensen, C E (1984). *Microalbuminuria predicts clinical proteinuria and early mortality in maturity onset diabetes.* New England Journal of Medicine 310:356-60.

Murphy, R P; Nanda, M; Plotnick, L; Enger, C; Vitale, S and Patz, A (1990). *The relationship of puberty to diabetic retinopathy.* Arch Ophthalmology 108:215-18.

Ryder, R E J; Dent, M T; Ward, J D (1992). *Testing for diabetic neuropathy, part two, autonomic neuropathy.* Practical Diabetes Vol 9; No 2:56-60.

Stamler, I; Rhomberg, P; Schoenberger, J A et al (1975). *Multi-variate analysis of the relationship of seven variables to blood pressure. Findings of the Chicago Heart Association Detection Project in Industry 1962-1972.* Journal of Chronic Disease 28:527-48.

Watkins, P J (1988). *ABC of Diabetes.* British Medical Journal.

Watkins, P J; Drury, P L; Taylor, K W (1990). *Diabetes and its Management.* Blackwell Scientific Publications.

Williams, J G (1991). *Diabetic autonomic neuropathy.* Practical Diabetes Vol 2; No 2:4-5.

Working Group on Hypertension and Diabetes (1987). *Statements on hypertension and diabetes: final report.* Arch Int Med 147:830-42.

23 Conclusion

In order to achieve the standard and quality of health care for people with diabetes outlined in the St Vincent Declaration, serious consideration must be given to the following:

- Continuing the search for information about the diabetes population.
- Improved information systems, in order to monitor the progress, effectiveness and outcome of diabetes education and care.
- Increased awareness, training and continuing education in diabetes care and management for all health care professionals.
- Support and training in the organisational and 'teaching' aspects of diabetes care in the primary health setting.
- Education for people with diabetes in the organisational aspects of their own care.
- Fostering of good working relationships between hospital diabetes teams and teams in general practice.
- Improved communication between hospital and general practice.
- Provision of care and the concept of 'shared' care clearly understood.
- Promotion of shared information about diabetes.
- Fostering general public knowledge of diabetes.

Living with diabetes is not easy and is not helped by the mystery, fear, judgement and stigma that even now surround this complex condition.

Providing diabetes care in general practice is a challenge, for it encompasses at least 50% of care for people with diabetes in the United Kingdom.

The primary care team is well placed to work towards achieving the goals set in the St Vincent Declaration 'to reduce the burden of diabetes for all'.

Appendices

I British Diabetic Association – unit membership for general practice

As part of the BDA's initiatives for primary health care there is a new professional membership category – unit membership for general practice.

This new category is a part of the Education and Professional Care Section and will come into effect on 1 June 1993.

Unit membership is open to a general practice but the name or title of an individual from the practice will be requested to whom information from the BDA might be sent. (Only one set of information will be sent to the practice at each mailing.)

The annual subscription is currently £15.00 and an information pack will be sent to all new unit members upon enrolment.

Unit membership will entitle a practice to one vote at an annual general meeting. However, if more than one individual from a practice which has membership wishes to attend an EPCS conference, all the individuals will pay the members' registration rate rather than the non-member's rate.

If you or any of your general practice colleagues would like forms, please send your request in *writing* to:

The Conference Office
British Diabetic Association
10 Queen Anne Street
London W1M 0BD

App I

II The rights and roles of people with diabetes – 'what care to expect'

The St Vincent Declaration implementation document provides a guideline for people with diabetes. This guideline is reflected in the British Diabetic Association leaflet *'Diabetes care – what you should expect'*, available FREE on request from the British Diabetic Association, 10 Queen Anne Street, London W1M 0BD. Telephone: 071 323 1531.

For all people with diabetes

Your guide to better diabetes care: rights and roles

A person with diabetes can, in general, lead a normal healthy and long life. Looking after yourself (self care) by learning about your diabetes provides the best chance to do this. Your doctor and other members of the health care team are there to advise you and to provide the information, support and technology so that you can look after yourself and live your life in the way you choose.

It is important that you know

1. What should be available from your health care providers to help you achieve these goals and
2. What *you* should do.

Your rights
The health care team (providers) should provide:

- a treatment plan and self care targets
- regular checks of blood sugar (glucose) levels
- regular checks of your physical condition
- treatment for special problems and emergencies
- continuing education for you and your family
- information on available social and economic support

Your role is
- to build this advice into your daily life
- to be in control of your diabetes on a day to day basis

Continuing Education

The following are important items you should learn about:

1. Why to control blood glucose levels.
2. How to control your blood glucose levels through proper eating, physical activity, tablets and/or insulin.
3. How to monitor your control with blood or urine tests (self-monitoring) and how to act on the results.
4. The signs of low and high blood glucose levels and ketosis, how to treat these conditions and how to prevent them.
5. What to do when you are ill.
6. The possible long term complications – including possible damage to eyes, nerves, kidneys and feet and hardening of the arteries; their prevention and treatment.
7. How to deal with lifestyle variations such as exercise, travelling and social activities, including drinking alcohol.
8. How to handle possible problems with employment, insurance, driving licences etc (see *Note* at end of this chapter).

Treatment plan and self care targets

The following should be given to you:

1. Personalised advice on proper eating – types of food, amounts and timing
2. Advice on physical activity
3. Your dose and timing of tablets or insulin and how to take them; advice on how to change doses based on your self-monitoring
4. Your target values for blood glucose, blood fats, blood pressure and weight.

Regular assessment

App II

The following should be done at each visit to your health care professionals. (NB These may vary according to your particular needs).

1. Review of your self-monitoring results and current treatment.
2. Talk about your targets and change where necessary.
3. Talk about any problems and questions you may have.
4. Continued education.

The health care team should check:

1. Your blood glucose control by taking special blood tests such as those for glycosylated haemoglobin, fructosamine or fasting blood glucose in non-insulin treated people. These can be done two to four times a year if your diabetes is well controlled.
2. Your weight.
3. Your blood pressure and blood fats if necessary.

The following should be checked at least once per year:

1. Your vision and eyes (with dilated pupils)
2. Your kidney function (blood and urine tests)
3. Your feet
4. Your risk factors for heart disease, such as blood pressure, blood fats and smoking habits
5. Your self-monitoring and injection techniques
6. Your eating habits.

Special problems

1. Advice and care should be available if you are planning to become pregnant
2. The needs of children and adolescents should be cared for
3. If you have problems with eyes, kidneys, feet, blood vessels or heart you should be able to see specialists quickly
4. In the elderly strict treatment is often unnecessary, you may want to discuss this with your health care team
5. The first months after your diabetes has been discovered are often difficult. Remember you cannot learn everything during this period – learning will continue for the rest of your life.

Your role
- Take control of your diabetes on a day to day basis. This will be easier the more you know about diabetes
- Learn about and practice self care. This includes monitoring glucose levels and how to change your treatment according to the results
- Examine your feet regularly
- Follow good lifestyle practices. These include choosing the right food, weight control, regular physical activity and not smoking
- Know when to contact your health care team urgently, especially in an emergency
- Talk regularly with your health care team about questions and concerns you may have

- Ask questions and repeat them if you are still unclear. Prepare your questions beforehand
- Speak to your health care team, other people with diabetes and your local or national diabetes associations and read pamphlets and books about diabetes, provided by your health care team or diabetes association. Make sure your family and friends know about the needs of your diabetes.

If you feel that adequate facilities and care are not available to help you look after your diabetes, contact your local or national diabetes association.

Note
'The St Vincent Declaration seeks to promote independence, equity and self-sufficiency for people with diabetes and the removal of hindrances to their full integration into society'

For example:

Driving licences
'Prejudice should not prevent diabetic people whose disease is well controlled and who have satisfactory vision from driving cars or certain other types of vehicle. Steps should be taken to remove any unreasonable restrictions.'

Employment
'Nearly all people with diabetes are capable of working as well as their non-diabetic fellows. Exceptions to this rule are very few. Steps should be taken to remove ignorance and prejudice in this area.'

Insurance
'Although the position has improved considerably in Denmark, France, Italy and the United Kingdom, the word must be spread that diabetic people who properly monitor their disease have a near normal life expectancy and should therefore not be asked to pay heavy premiums for life or health insurance. Improvements are also needed in both motor and travel insurance.'

The leaflet *Your guide to better diabetes care: rights and roles* is available from Boehringer Mannheim UK (see resources list chapter 16).

App II

III St Vincent Declaration recommendations for the care of children

These are the St Vincent Declaration recommendations for the care of children and adolescents with diabetes.

Diagnosis

"Early symptoms of diabetes in children and adolescents (such as thirst, increased urine production and weight loss) should be made familiar not only to all health care professionals but also to the general population. Information about diabetes should be spread through the mass media and included in school curricula. Test materials for the measurement of glucose in urine should be available to all health care professionals."

Treatment

"Newly diagnosed patients should be treated at units whose staff have specialised knowledge of diabetes in children and adolescents. The diabetes care team should include a paediatric diabetologist, a dietitian, a specialist diabetes nurse and a social worker or psychologist.

Long term care should be managed by a paediatrician experienced in the care of diabetic children. The interval between follow up visits should be one to three months, but shorter when needed: for example after major treatment adjustments. Long term glucose control should be estimated by measurement of glycosylated haemoglobin at least every three months. Growth and pubertal development should be followed regularly and values plotted on growth charts. The general practitioner can handle some acute problems and under exceptional circumstances intermediate consultation but always in consultation with the responsible diabetologist."

Recommendations

Recommendations are made for a standard of care for children and adolescents. They include – education appropriate to age and including the family, school or college. This education should be provided orally and in writing and should encompass information about weekends, holidays and camps.

Fig III.I Examples of St Vincent Declaration leaflets.

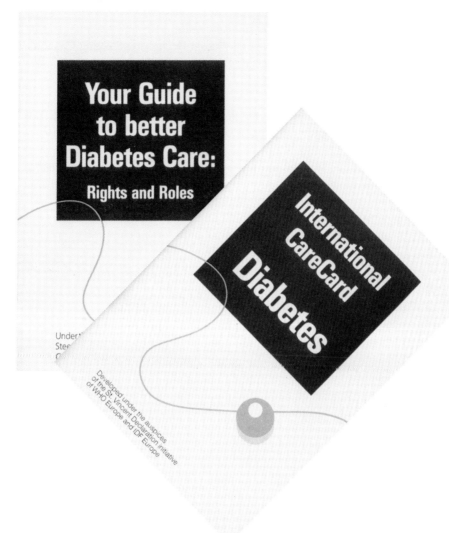

Recommendations for specialist teams also include:-

Psychological/social support
Insulin treatment
Nutrition
Self-management
Blood glucose control – targets
Late vascular complications
Social rights

Information

Your guide to better diabetes care: right and roles
Produced under the auspices of the St Vincent Declaration Steering Committee of IDF/WHO Europe and the Council of the European Region of the IDF.

International care card: diabetes
Developed under the auspices of the St Vincent Declaration initiative of WHO Europe and IDF Europe.

Both these cards (see Fig III.I) are sponsored by Boehringer Mannheim UK and are available on application from:

Boehringer Mannheim UK
(Diagnostics and Biochemicals) Limited
Bell Lane
Lewes
East Sussex
BN7 1LG
Telephone: 0273 480444
Fax: 0273 480266

IV Department of Health requirements

The outline arrangements for diabetes in general practice are as follows:

Aims, responsibilities and educational needs relating to existing and new arrangements

New arrangements for banded/costed health promotion clinics reflect objectives set out in the *Health of the Nation*. Initially, they will focus on three main areas – smoking cessation, coronary heart disease and stroke. The Department of Health expects general practitioners to run disease management programmes for asthma and diabetes, each attracting an annual allowance for general practitioners involved in the schemes

Practices must set up an organised programme for the care of patients with diabetes mellitus

What practices have to do
- Keep an up to date register of all patients with diabetes
- Ensure a systematic call and recall of patients on this register is taking place either to hospital or the practice
- Provide education for newly diagnosed diabetics, ensuring that all newly diagnosed patients and/or their carers receive appropriate education and advice on the management and prevention of secondary complications of their diabetes
- Ensure that all patients with diabetes or their carers receive continuing education
- Ensure that at initial diagnosis and at least annually, a full review of the patient's health is carried out including checks for potential complications and a review of the patient's own monitoring records
- Prepare an individual management plan with the patient
- Work together with other professionals such as dietitians and chiropodists and ensure that they are appropriately trained in the management of diabetes

App IV

217

- Refer patients to secondary care where appropriate and to relevant support agencies
- Maintain adequate records of performance and results of these procedures, including information from other people involved in the care of patients
- Audit the care of patients with diabetes against the above criteria.

Practices approved for chronic disease management have to include reports on the progress of the programme and a summary of any clinical audit that has been carried out so far. They will have to provide numbers of their diabetic patients and include details of any treatment given or interventions made.

In-year monitoring
Practices accepted onto the banding scheme will have to produce a mini report covering the first six months of the scheme, from 1 July to 31 December 1993. If the practice plans any changes to its programmes it will have to say so in this report.

Practices must also include the numbers of patients already seen under the new health promotion and asthma and diabetes management programmes.

General practitioners not approved for any health promotion band.
Practices must still record numbers of patients who are smoking regularly; drinking more than the weekly amounts of alcohol liable to damage health; overweight and obese patients; asthmatics; diabetics.

Reference

NHS Management Executive. 12/01/93 GP contract health promotion package guidance on implementation.

V British Diabetic Association recommendations for the management of diabetes in primary care

British Diabetic Association recommendations (1993) for the management of diabetes in primary care are as follows.

Aims

The overall aim of any system of diabetes care is to produce a sustained improvement in the health of people with diabetes, resulting in a life approaching normal expectations, both in quality and duration.

It is generally believed that the maintenance of near normal blood glucose levels is the key, not only to avoiding the acute metabolic crises of hypoglycaemia and ketoacidosis but also to prevent the development of long-term complications. Attention to associated cardiovascular risk factors, including hyperlipidaemia and hypertension, is also important.

Behaviour modification through education together with regular monitoring of blood glucose control and appropriate management, are essential to the improvement of the health of people with diabetes. Increasingly it has been realised that the person with diabetes plays a crucial role in this process, and hence adequate motivation is essential. This education should be matched to the patient's ability and capacity to learn.

There is evidence that early treatment of many established complications can reduce morbidity and costs. In retinopathy, for example, the detection of early retinal disease followed by laser treatment can prevent blindness. Planned follow up with effective surveillance for complications is therefore essential.

People with diabetes should be empowered to obtain the maximum benefit from health care services so that they are able to participate in most activities open to those without diabetes.

App V

Objectives

The main objectives of diabetes care are therefore to ensure:

1. The provision of appropriate education to enable all people with diabetes to acquire the necessary knowledge and skills to take responsibility for managing their own health care, and to modify their lifestyle in such a way as to maximise their well being.
2. The maintenance of blood glucose control at as near physiological levels as possible, while at the same time aiming to achieve as near normal a lifestyle as possible, through regular monitoring of metabolic control and appropriate   management, thereby minimising the likelihood of people with diabetes developing short term and long term complications.
3. The identification and appropriate management of individuals with cardiovascular risk factors, including:

- smoking
- hyperlipidaemia
- hypertension

4. The early identification and appropriate management of individuals with long term complications of diabetes, in order to reduce:

- angina and myocardial infarction
- foot ulceration and limb amputation due to peripheral vascular disease and diabetic neuropathy
- blindness and visual impairment resulting from diabetic retinopathy
- stroke and other cerebrovascular disease
- end-stage renal failure due to diabetic nephropathy

5. The strict maintenance of blood glucose control before conception and throughout pregnancy in diabetic women in order to reduce foetal loss during pregnancy, still-births and congenital malformations and neonatal problems in the children of mothers with diabetes.

Purpose

The British Diabetic Association (BDA) has recently produced a leaflet for people with diabetes entitled *Diabetes Care – what you should expect*. The leaflet, which is available from the BDA, explains what treatment and advice patients should expect from their health care team.

The leaflet stresses the importance of patients understanding their diabetes so that they are enabled to become effective members of the health care team. Increasingly, patients will therefore expect to receive the level of care specified in the leaflet, whether their diabetes care is being provided in a hospital or primary care setting.

It is the GP who has overall responsibility for ensuring that all registered patients with diabetes are involved in a planned programme of diabetes care.

The first step to achieving this aim is to identify all registered patients with diagnosed diabetes. This will involve the setting up and maintenance of a practice register of patients with diabetes, which should ideally be computerised and possibly linked to a district diabetes register.

Patients can then be categorised according to where their planned programme of care is being provided.

The appropriate setting for the various elements of a programme of diabetes care will vary according to the needs of the particular patient. It will be for the GP, in consultation with members of the hospital diabetes team, to decide where a particular patient receives each element of care.

It is essential for the GP to provide planned follow up for any patient not receiving such care elsewhere. The components of the management plan should be discussed and agreed with each individual patient. A patient held record card can facilitate this process.

A planned programme of diabetes care must include the following elements:

- assessment and initial management of newly diagnosed and rediscovered patients
- initial stabilisation and education of these patients
- regular review and maintenance of metabolic control
- regular review and management of cardiovascular risk factors
- on-going education
- management of acute complications
- detection and management of long term complications

Patients within certain agreed groups will need to be followed up by the   hospital diabetes team. These will usually include:

- all children and adolescents
- all patients considering pregnancy or who are already pregnant
- all patients with significant complications

App V

In many localities, the majority of insulin treated patients will also be followed up in the hospital setting. Referral should also be considered of patients with unsatisfactory metabolic or blood pressure control.

In order to meet the needs of all patients with diagnosed diabetes there should be integrated primary and hospital based care. Ideally, district diabetes policies should be agreed with set out referral criteria for patients with diabetes, including the timing and route of such referrals. Such criteria must also take account of the different levels of skill and interest in the management of diabetes amongst primary health care teams. Following discussion, it may be decided that some patients, currently being followed up in the hospital setting, could in future either be followed up by the primary health care team, or be the subject of shared care between the primary care and hospital based diabetes teams.

Reference

British Diabetic Association. Diabetes Services Advisory Committee (1993). *Recommendations for the management of diabetes in primary care.*

Index

acromegaly 192
action
  biguanides 84, 180
  insulin preparations 90
  sulphonylureas 82, 180
activity for health 81
acute glaucoma 127
acute outcomes 166
addresses, useful
  BDA 173, 209
  companies 174-5, 199, 216
  insurance brokers 176
  miscellaneous organisations 176
  publishers 171-2, 174
  travel and holidays 163
administering insulin *see*
    insulin injections;
    insulin pumps
administrative staff 7-8, 53
adolescents *see* young people
Afro-Caribbeans, prevalence of
    NIDDM 17
age, effect on
  diabetic retinopathy 17, 200
  feet 131
  glycaemic control targets 66
  prevalence of diabetes 16-17
  renal threshold 49, 116

aims
  BDA recommendations for
    management of diabetes in
    primary care 219
  care provision 21
  insulin therapy for NIDDM 88
  practice diabetes register 55
  practice diabetes service 33
  St Vincent Declaration xi-xii
  treatment of NIDDM 72-4, 186
alcohol
  BDA recommendations 79-80
  drug interactions 87
  key information points for patient
    education 156
annual reports, FHSA requirements
    169-70
annual reviews 67
  assessment of self management 147
  key information points for patient
    education 156-7
antenatal care, gestational diabetes
    190
appointments, time needed 37, 68
Asians
  BDA dietary recommendations 80,
    104
  languages 104

Asians *(continued)*
    prevalence of diabetes 17, 99, 185
    prevalence of microalbuminuria
        198
    religions and culture 99-105
assessments
    candidates for insulin therapy 92
    candidates for self management 147
    newly diagnosed patients 61-4, 147
    rights and roles of people with
        diabetes 211-12
    for self monitoring 113
atherosclerosis 203
attitudes, to diabetes 144-7
audits *see* clinical audit and evaluation;
        monitoring and audit
autonomic neuropathy 197, 202
    effect on feet 131-2

background retinopathy 197, 200-1
Balance 28, 173
Balance for Beginners 28, 173
basement membrane, effect of
        diabetes 196
BDA
    address 173, 209
    booklets and leaflets 173, 210, 220
    clinical audit and evaluation guide
        lines 165-8
    dietary recommendations 79-80,
        104
    dietitians 28, 104
    as information source 28, 29, 173
    organisation and roles 27-9
    recommendations for the manage-
        ment of diabetes in primary care
        219-22
    St Vincent declaration joint
        DOH/BDA task force xiii
    unit membership for general
        practice 209
beef insulin 89, 90

beliefs
    Hindu 100
    Islam 101
    Sikhs 102
biguanides 82, 84-5, 180
    see also metformin
biosynthetic insulins 89
blindness, statistics 17, 201
blood glucose levels
    control of *see* monitoring and
        control
    fasting *see* fasting blood glucose
        levels
    high *see* hyperglycaemia
    low *see* hypoglycaemia
    measuring equipment 40-1,
        117-18
    monitoring *see* monitoring and
        control
    random *see* random blood glucose
        levels
blood glucose meters 41, 118
blood pressure
    control postpones diabetic
        nephropathy 199
    hypertension 203, 204
    key information points for patient
        education 156
blood testing
    at annual reviews 67
    at initial assessment 62
    at routine reviews 66
    equipment 40-1, 117-18
    key information points for patient
        education 155
    self monitoring 116-18, 183
    techniques 117
BMI 61, 75
body mass index *see* BMI
booklets and leaflets 42
    from BDA 173, 210, 220
    insulin therapy 94

booklets and leaflets *(continued)*
  rights and roles of people with
    diabetes 210, 213, 215, 216
  St Vincent Declaration leaflets
    215, 216
  urine testing for glycosuria 115
books
  for patients 171-2
  for primary care team 172
branches, BDA 28-9, 57
breast screening 159
British Diabetic Association *see* BDA

calories, BDA recommendations 79
candidates
  assessment of candidates for self
    management 147
  for foot problems 135-6
  for insulin therapy 92
  for practice diabetes register 53-5
  for screening 48
capillary blood testing, equipment 40-1
carbohydrates
  BDA recommendations 79, 181
  emergency exchange list 110-11
carcinoma of the pancreas 192
cardiovascular disease 73, 197, 203,
    204
  see also heart attacks and heart
    disease
cardiovascular risk factors, outcome
    measures 167
care provision
  aims 21
  BDA recommendations for the
    management of diabetes in
    primary care 219-22
  for children 21, 23
  in diabetes centres 26-7
  in hospital clinics 21-2
  key information points for patient
    education 153

care provision *(continued)*
  organisation in UK 21-9
  recorded in practice diabetes
    register 56
  role of BDA 27-9
  statistics 21-2
  variation in standards of care 21
  see also practice diabetes service;
    responsibilities for care provi-
    sion; roles in care provision
cataracts 127, 197, 203
causes
  complications of diabetes 196
  of diabetes, hereditary 193-4
  of diabetes, hormonal 192
  foot ulceration 131-3
  hyperglycaemia 107-8
  hypoglycaemia 90-1, 96, 111
  IDDM 183
  secondary diabetes 192-5
cervical screening 159
children
  care provision 21, 23
  diabetes clinics 21, 61
  diabetic retinopathy 200
  key information points for patient
    education 159-60
  prevalence of diabetes 17
  St Vincent Declaration recommen-
    dations 214-16
  services from BDA 28
chiropodists
  establishing availability of services
    58
  key information points for patient
    education 157
  referral for foot ulceration 143
  roles in care provision 25-6
  State Registered 25, 26
cholesterol levels, testing 62, 67
chronic glaucoma 127
circulation, abnormal *see* ischaemia

classification, diabetes 179
clerical staff 7-8, 53
clinical audit and evaluation
    BDA guidelines 165-8
    computer programs 169
    measures of health status, quality of
        life and patient satisfaction 167
    minimum dataset 168
    outcome measures 166-7
    process measures 166
clinical management
    diabetes 61-71
    foot ulceration 142-3
    gestational diabetes 190
    hyperglycaemia 108
    intercurrent illnesses 108
    newly diagnosed patients 61-4
    normal weight patients 64, 81
    overweight patients 63, 75, 80-1
    see also protocols; treatment
clinics see diabetes clinics; hospital
    clinics
closed angle glaucoma 127
co-ordinating function
    practice nurses 5
    role of diabetes centres 27
codes of conduct 3
colour vision test cards 123
combination therapy 86, 186
community dietitians 24-5, 76
community nurses, educational courses
    available 11-12
company addresses 174-5, 199, 216
complications of diabetes 17-21,
    196-205
    causes 196
    criteria for hospital referral 65
    effect of duration of diabetes 196,
        200, 203
    effect on feet 131-3
    fear of 145
    investigating at annual reviews 67

complications of diabetes (continued)
    investigating at initial assessment
        62
    long term, statistics 196
    markers of late complications 167
    patterns of association 196
    prevention 73-4
    recorded in practice diabetes
        register 56
    see also individually by type
        eg diabetic retinopathy
computer programs, clinical audit and
    evaluation 169
conception, key information points
    for patient education 158
consequences of diabetes 18-21
    see also individually by type
        eg strokes
contact lens fitters 125
contact names and numbers
    key information points for patient
        education 154
    for patients on insulin 96
    specialist and support services 42,
        56-7
contact with patients, practice nurses
    4
contraception, key information points
    for patient education 157-8
contraindications
    guar gum 86
    metformin 85
    sulphonylureas 84
coronary artery disease see cardio-
    vascular disease
costs of diabetes 20-1
courses, for primary care team 11-12
cranial nerve palsies 197
crb insulin 89
criteria
    clinical audit and evaluation 165
    hospital referral 61, 65

criteria (*continued*)
　referral of foot ulceration to
　　specialist services 142-3
cultural factors 99-105, 144-5
Cushing's syndrome 192
cystic fibrosis 192

dark rooms 38
data, minimum dataset for diabetes
　management 168
dental care, key information points for
　patient education 164
Department of Health *see* DOH
diabetes
　attitudes of patients and families
　　144-7
　classification and types 179
　clinical management 61-71
　complications *see* complications of
　　diabetes
　consequences *see* consequences of
　　diabetes
　costs 20-1
　diagnosis 49-52
　drug-induced 193
　effect on basement membrane 196
　hereditary causes 193-4
　history 179-81
　hormonal causes 192
　organs affected 196
　patient's knowledge of diabetes
　　47-8, 153
　prevalence 16-17, 54
　public awareness 47-8
　screening 40, 48
　secondary 192-5
　treatment *see* treatment of diabetes
　visual changes during stabilisation
　　120-1
　see also by type eg IDDM
diabetes care provision *see* care provi-
　sion; practice diabetes service

diabetes centres 26-7
diabetes clinics 21-2, 35
　see also hospital clinics; practice
　　diabetes service
diabetes insipidus 180
diabetes mellitus *see* diabetes
diabetes record cards 43-4
diabetes registers
　district 26, 165
　in practice diabetes service *see*
　　practice diabetes registers
diabetic foods, BDA recommend-
　ations 80
diabetic glomerulosclerosis 197
diabetic ketosis, prevalence 19-20
diabetic nephropathy 197-200
　delaying progression 198-9, 200
　prevalence 17-18, 197, 199
　progression 198
　symptoms 198
　see also renal failure
diabetic neuropathy 202-3
　effect on feet 131-3, 136
　prevalence 18, 202, 203
　see also autonomic neuropathy;
　　peripheral neuropathy
diabetic retinopathy 197, 200-2
　in children 200
　effectiveness of early treatment 20
　laser therapy 129, 201, 202
　patient care at detection 128
　peripheral maculopathy 126, 200-1
　prevalence 17, 200, 201
　prevention 201
　rate of onset 200, 201
　testing for *see* fundoscopy
　see also by type eg background
　　retinopathy
diabetologists 23
diagnosis
　clinical management of newly diag-
　　nosed patients 61-4

diagnosis (*continued*)
   of diabetes 49-52
   gestational diabetes 190
   IDDM 182
   NIDDM 185-6
dialysis 197, 198, 199, 200
DIDMOAD syndrome 193
diet
   emergency exchange list 110-11
   Hindus 100
   hot and cold foods 102-4
   Moslems 101
   Sikhs 102
   see also dietary recommendations
      and treatment
dietary recommendations and treatment
   75-81, 186
   BDA recommendations 79-80, 104
   emergency exchange list 110-11
   gestational diabetes 190
   healthy eating 76-80
   history 180-1
   key information points for patient
      education 153
   normal weight patients 81
   overweight patients 80-1
   protein restriction in IDDM 199,
      200
   roles of dietitians 24-5, 75-6
dietitians
   BDA 28, 104
   establishing availability of services
      57
   roles in care provision 24-5, 75-6
dispensing opticians 125
distance learning courses 12
distance vision testing 123
District Health Authorities, provision
   of chiropody services 25
DOH
   monitoring and audit requirements
      218

DOH (*continued*}
   practice diabetes register require-
      ments 55, 217
   practice diabetes service requirements
      217-18
   prescription exemption forms 82,
      154
   St Vincent declaration joint
      DOH/BDA task force xiii
drawing up insulin 94
driving and driving licences 161-2,
   186, 213
drug interactions 87, 193
   key information points for patient
      education 155
drug treatment 75, 82-6, 87, 186
   key information points for patient
      education 154
drug-induced diabetes 193
DVLC 161-2

eating
   eating out, key information points
      for patient education 156
   healthy 76-80
education
   affecting self-management ability
      145
   courses for GPs 12
   courses for nurses 11-12
   needs, administrative staff 8
   needs, primary care team 9-15
   of patients *see* patient education
   self-help, primary care team 12
   syllabus for primary care team
      13-15
effectiveness, of treatment for
   diabetes 20
emp insulin 89
employment
   affecting self-management ability
      146

employment (*continued*)
key information points for patient
education 160
St Vincent Declaration recommendations 213
English National Board for Nursing,
Midwifery and Health Visiting
11, 175
equipment
blood glucose measurement 41
blood testing 40-1, 117-18
clinical management of hyperglycaemia 108
foot examination 133-4
fundoscopy 38, 41, 126
glycosuria testing 40
insulin therapy 93-4, 95
ketonuria testing 40
microalbuminuria testing 40, 198,
199
OGTT 40
peripheral neuropathy testing 41
practice diabetes service 39 41
proteinuria testing 40, 198
screening 40
urine testing 40
visual acuity testing 41, 121-3
see also materials and resources
evaluation
clinical audit *see* clinical audit and
evaluation
group education sessions 150-1
patient education 97-8
self monitoring 114
examinations *see* reviews; screening;
tests
exercise and sport 81, 160-1, 185
eye care and screening 119-29, 201, 202
free NHS eye tests 121, 127
key information points for patient
education 157
role of hospital clinics 119

eye care and screening (*continued*)
role of practice diabetes service 119
role of primary care team 119-20
see also individual disorders, tests
and treatments eg fundoscopy
eyes, temporary visual changes 120-1

facilities for practice diabetes service
38-9
Family Health Services Authority *see*
FHSA
family planning, key information points
for patient education 157-8
fasting blood glucose levels
compared to HbA_1 106
confirmation of diagnosis 49, 52,
186
glycaemic control targets 66
indicating IGT 51, 186
sign of diabetes 46
fats, BDA recommendations 79
feet
at risk 131 3, 135 6
diabetic 131-3
effect of age 131
ischaemic 133, 202, 203
neuropathic 133, 202, 203
non-diabetic 131
see also foot care and surveillance;
foot ulceration
festivals
Hindu 100
Islam 101
Sikhs 102
FHS Computer Unit 165, 169
FHSA, practice diabetes service
monitoring requirements 169-70
flexibility, practice nurses 6
follow up and recall 67-70
foods
diabetic 80
hot and cold 102-4

foods (*continued*)
　　see also diet; dietary recommend-
　　　ations and treatment
foot care and surveillance 130-43,
　　202, 203
　　equipment 133-4
　　identification of 'at risk' patients
　　　135-6
　　patient education 136-41, 157
　　protocols for foot, footwear and
　　　shoe examinations 134-5
　　roles of chiropodists 25
　　roles of hospital clinics 130
　　roles of practice diabetes service
　　　130
　　roles of primary care team 130-1
foot ulceration 18, 131-3, 142-3
footwear
　　examination 135
　　patient education 141
frequency, recall and follow up 68-9
funding, BDA 29
fundoscopy 126-8, 201, 202
　　by ophthalmic opticians 126
　　equipment 38, 41, 126
　　preparation of patient 126-7
　　protocol 127-8

General Medical Council 3
general practice
　　BDA initiatives 29
　　BDA unit membership 209
　　numbers of practice nurses 4
　　practice information 43-4
　　prevalence of diabetes 54
　　see also practice diabetes service;
　　　practice team
general practitioners *see* GPs
gestational diabetes 116, 179, 189-90
glaucoma 127
glomerular filtration rate 198
glucagon 41, 112-13, 192

glycaemic control targets 66
glycosuria
　　diagnosis of diabetes 49
　　sign of diabetes 46
　　testing materials 40, 115-16
　　see also renal threshold; urine
　　　testing
glycosylated haemoglobin 106
GPs
　　choice of GPs to be involved in
　　　practice diabetes service 36-7
　　clinical management of hypergly-
　　　caemia 108
　　educational courses 12
　　responsibilities for care provision
　　　3
　　responsibilities as employers 3
group education sessions 148-52
guar gum 82, 86

haemochromatosis 192-3
HbA$_1$ 106
healthy eating 76-80
heart attacks and heart disease,
　　prevalence 19, 203
hearty breakfast test 51
high renal threshold 49-50
Hindus 100, 104
history, diabetes 179-81
holidays *see* travel and holidays
hormone replacement therapy, key
　　information points for patient
　　education 158
hospital clinics 21-2, 26
　　eye care and screening provisions
　　　119
　　foot care and surveillance
　　　provisions 130
　　referral for foot ulceration 142
　　see also diabetes centres; diabetes
　　　clinics
hospital referral, criteria 61, 65

HRT, key information points for patient education 158
human insulin 89, 91, 180
hyperglycaemia 73, 107-8, 182-3
  factor in cardiovascular disease 203, 204
  key information points for patient education 155
hypertension 203, 204
hypoglycaemia 111-13, 186
  causes 96, 111, 182
  diminished warning signs 91, 112
  effect of change of insulin 90-1
  emergency treatment materials 41
  patient education 96, 154
  prevention 73, 96
  symptoms 112
  treatment 96, 112-13
hypoglycaemic agents, oral see oral hypoglycaemic agents
Hypostop gel 41, 112

IDDM 182-4
  causes 183
  classification 179, 180
  compared to NIDDM 187
  diagnosis 182
  hyperglycaemia 182-3
  hypertension 203, 204
  hypoglycaemia 182
  long term complications 196
  prevalence 16-17, 183
  protein restriction in diet 199, 200
  referral to diabetes centres 61, 65, 75
  self monitoring 115, 116, 183
  signs 46
  symptoms 45-6, 182
  symptoms of diabetic nephropathy 198
  treatment 182
identification cards and jewellery 42, 97

IGT 51, 179, 186, 189
illness
  illness rules in NIDDM 109, 155
  intercurrent see intercurrent illnesses
impaired glucose tolerance see IGT
impotence 18, 159, 202
in-year monitoring, FHSA requirements 169
incidence see prevalence
indemnity, practice nurses 3
influenza vaccination 159
information
  key information points for living with diabetes 153-64
  for patients see patient education
  practice see practice information
  recording see record keeping
  see also by type of information required eg addresses, useful
information requirements
  availability of specialist services 42, 56-8
  availability of support services 42, 60
  BDA as information source 28, 29, 173
  clinical audit and evaluation 165-70
  materials and resources for patient education 42, 148, 171-6
  minimum dataset for diabetes management 168
initial assessments, newly diagnosed patients 61-4, 147
injection sites 90, 95
injections, insulin see insulin injections
insulin
  benefits 92
  discovery 180
  sources 89

insulin (*continued*)
  types of preparation available 90
  see also by type eg human insulin
insulin dependent diabetes *see* IDDM
insulin injections 89-90
  booklets and leaflets 94
  drawing up dose 94
  dummy injections 92
  equipment 93-4, 95
  giving the injection 95
  injection sites 90, 95
  key information points for patient
    education 154
  patient education for self adminis-
    tration 91-8
  patients' problems and questions
    97
  see also pen devices; syringes
insulin pumps 90
insulin therapy for NIDDM 86-98,
    186
  administering insulin *see* insulin
    injections; insulin pumps
  aims 88
  assessing candidates for self admin-
    istration 92
  booklets and leaflets 94
  changing insulins 90-1
  criteria 86-8
  during intercurrent illnesses 88
  key information points for patient
    education 154
  loss of vocational driving licences
    161-2, 186
  side effects *see* hypoglycaemia
  starting treatment 88
  trial period 88, 186
insurance 162
  brokers 176
  St Vincent Declaration recommen-
    dations 213
integrated courses 11-12

intercurrent illnesses
  clinical management 108
  criteria for insulin therapy for
    NIDDM 86-8
  illness rules in NIDDM 109, 155
intermediate outcomes 167
international care cards 215, 216
ischaemia
  effect on feet 131-3, 135, 202,
    203
  prevalence 19
Islam 101
islet cell tumours 193

journals, for primary care team 174

ketonuria
  criteria for hospital referral 61, 65
  criteria for insulin therapy for
    NIDDM 86-7
  sign of diabetes 46
  testing equipment 40
ketosis *see* diabetic ketosis
kidney failure *see* renal failure
knowledge about diabetes
  among general public 47
  self-assessment for primary care
    team 9-10

languages
  avoiding medical terminology
    146
  Hindus 104
  Indo-Asian 104
  Moslems 104
  need for translators 145
  Sikhs 104
laser therapy 17, 129, 201, 202
late outcomes 167
leaflets *see* booklets and leaflets
leisure activities *see* social life; sport
    and exercise; travel and holidays

letters
  advertising the practice diabetes
    service 59, 60
  invitation to group education session 149
licences, driving 161-2, 186, 213
life insurance 162
  brokers 176
lifestyles
  affecting self-management ability 146-7
  ensuring satisfactory lifestyle 72
literacy levels, affecting self-management ability 145
low renal threshold 49-50

malnutrition related diabetes mellitus 179, 194
management *see* clinical management; self management
materials and resources
  clinical management of hyperglycaemia 108
  emergency hypoglycaemia treatment 41
  patient education 42, 148, 171-6
  record keeping 42-3
  see also equipment
mature onset diabetes of the young *see* MODY
measures
  health status, quality of life and patient satisfaction 167
  outcome 166-7
  process 166
Medical Audit Advisory Groups 165
Medical Defence Union 3
medication *see* drug treatment; oral hypoglycaemic agents
membership, BDA 27, 209
mental difficulties, affecting self-management ability 145

metformin 85, 86, 87
microalbuminuria 198, 199
  testing equipment 40, 198, 199
MODY 185, 194
monitoring and audit
  BDA guidelines 165-8
  DOH requirements 218
  FHSA requirements 169-70
  practice diabetes service 165-70
monitoring and control 98, 106-18
  benefits 106-7
  glycaemic control targets 66
  hyperglycaemia 108
  key information points for patient education 155
  in pregnancy 183
  reasons for 114-15
  role in postponing diabetic nephropathy 199
  role of primary care team 106-7
  self monitoring 113-18, 183
  see also individual tests by type eg serum fructosamine
mortality, deaths due to diabetes 18-19
Moslems 101, 104
mydriatic drops 126, 127-8

National Health Service *see* NHS
near vision test cards 122
needle clippers 93
nephropathy *see* diabetic nephropathy
nephrotic syndrome 198
neuropathy *see* diabetic neuropathy
NHS
  costs of diabetes 20-1
  free eye tests 121, 127
NIDDM 185-8
  aims of treatment 72-4, 186
  blood testing 116-17
  classification 179, 180
  compared to IDDM 187

NIDDM (*continued*)

complications *see* complications of diabetes

diagnosis 185-6

dietary treatment 75-81, 186

drug treatment 75, 82-6, 87, 154, 186

hypertension 203, 204

illness rules 109, 155

insulin therapy 86-98, 186

prevalence 16-17, 22, 185

prevalence of microalbuminuria 198

protocols for diagnosis and management 63-4

research projects 27

signs 46

starting treatment 74-5

symptoms 45-6, 72, 186

symptoms of diabetic nephropathy 198

undiagnosed 17, 45, 47, 185, 196

urine testing 115-16

non-insulin dependent diabetes *see* NIDDM

normal weight patients

clinical management 64

dietary recommendations and treatment 81

nurse specialists, roles in care provision 23-4

nurses *see* by speciality eg practice nurses

nursing courses 11-12

objectives

BDA recommendations for the management of diabetes in primary care 220

practice diabetes service 33-4

OGTT

confirming diabetes diagnosis 49, 186

OGTT (*continued*)

confirming IGT 51

equipment 40

gestational diabetes 190

protocol 51-2

ophthalmic opticians 125-6

opportunities for screening 48

opticians 125-6

oral glucose tolerance test *see* OGTT

oral hypoglycaemic agents 82-6, 186

drug interactions 87

first production 180

key information points for patient education 154

see also by type eg biguanides

organisation

care provision in UK 21-9

group education sessions 148-52

options for practice diabetes service 35-6, 37-8

practice diabetes register 55-6

recall and follow up 67-70

record keeping 43-4

organs affected by diabetes 196

outcome measures 166-7

overweight patients

clinical management 63, 75

cultural factors 145

dietary recommendations and treatment 80-1

paediatricians 21, 23

pancreatic disease 192

pancreatitis 192

patient education

anticipating questions 97

contact telephone numbers 96, 154

in diabetes centres 26-7

DOH requirements 217

drug treatment 82, 154

emergency exchange list 110-11

evaluating 97-8, 150-1

patient education (*continued*)
  foot care and surveillance 136-41
  footwear advice 141
  getting the message across 148-52
  group sessions 148-52
  healthy eating 76-8
  hypoglycaemia 96
  illness rules 109, 155
  key information points 153-64
  laser therapy 129
  'learning', 'understanding' and 'doing' gaps 144-7
  problems in information giving 146
  psychological factors 144-7
  rights and roles of people with diabetes 211
  self administration of insulin 91-8
  for self management 144-52
  self monitoring 113-18
  shoe care and examination 139-40
  starting treatment for NIDDM 74-5
  see also booklets and leaflets; books; materials and resources
patients
  assessing candidates for insulin therapy 92
  assessing candidates for self management 147
  at diagnosis 49, 144
  candidates for foot problems 135-6
  candidates for practice diabetes register 53-5
  candidates for screening 48
  normal weight 64, 81
  overweight 63, 75, 80-1, 145
  patient satisfaction measures 167
  patients' records *see* record keeping
  personal contact by practice nurses 4
  preparation for fundoscopy 126-7
  requiring care at home 6, 35-6
  rights and roles 210-13

patients (*continued*)
  suitability for practice diabetes service 36
pen devices 89-90, 93
peripheral maculopathy 126, 200-1
peripheral mononeuropathy 197
peripheral neuropathy 197, 202
  effect on feet 131-2, 202, 203
  testing equipment 41
peripheral vascular disease *see* ischaemia
personal contact with patients, practice nurses 4
phaeochromocytoma 192
pharmaceutical company addresses 174-5, 199, 216
pharmacists 54
photocoagulation therapy *see* laser therapy
physical difficulties, affecting self-management ability 145
physicians *see* by speciality eg diabetologists
pinhole cards 41, 121-2, 123
planned courses 11-12
planning, practice diabetes service 34-9
podiatrists 25
pork insulin 89, 91
posters 42
  advertising practice diabetes service 58, 60
  diabetes symptoms 47
  foot care advice 137-8
  footwear advice 141
  healthy eating 77-8
  identifying diabetics 54
  shoe care and examination 139-40
postgraduate courses 12
practice diabetes registers
  aims 55
  DOH requirements 55, 217

practice diabetes registers *(continued)*
  example of register 57
  identifying candidates for register
    53-5
  patients with 'at risk' feet 135
  set-up and maintenance 55-6
practice diabetes service
  advertising the service 58-60
  aims 33
  availability 22
  BDA clinical audit and evaluation
    guidelines 165-8
  BDA recommendations for the
    management of diabetes in
    primary care 219-22
  DOH requirements 217-18
  equipment 39-41
  eye care and screening provisions
    119-20
  facilities 38-9
  FHSA monitoring requirements
    169-70
  foot care and surveillance
    provisions 130
  links with specialist teams 34, 36,
    56-7
  monitoring and audit 165-70
  objectives 33-4
  organisation options 35-6, 37-8
  planning 34-9
  recall and follow up 67-70
  recording information *see* record
    keeping
  register *see* practice diabetes
    registers
  role in achieving St Vincent
    Declaration targets 206
  roles of practice team 34-5, 36-7
  setting it up 33-44
  suitability of patients 36
practice information 43-4
practice managers 8

practice nurses
  co-ordinating function 5
  educational courses 11-12
  flexibility 6
  indemnity 3
  numbers in general practice 4
  responsibilities for care provision 3
  roles in care provision 4-6, 75
  roles in practice diabetes service 37
practice team
  roles in care provision 3-8
  roles in planning practice diabetes
    service 34-5
  roles in providing practice diabetes
    service 36-7
  see also individual members of
    team eg GPs; primary care team
prb insulin 89
pre-conception
  importance of monitoring and
    control 183
  key information points for patient
    education 158
pre-proliferative retinopathy 201
pregnancy
  blood testing 116, 183
  criteria for hospital referral 61, 65
  effect on renal threshold 49
  hot and cold foods 102
  hyperglycaemia 107
  key information points for patient
    education 158
  pregnancy outcomes 167
  risks 183, 190
  self monitoring 116, 183
  see also gestational diabetes
prescription exemption forms 82, 154
prevalence
  diabetes 16-17, 54
  diabetic ketosis 19-20
  diabetic nephropathy 17-18, 197,
    199

prevalence (*continued*)
   diabetic neuropathy 18, 202, 203
   diabetic retinopathy 17, 200, 201
   foot ulceration 18
   heart attacks and heart disease 19, 203
   IDDM 16-17, 183
   ischaemia 19
   microalbuminuria in NIDDM 198
   NIDDM 16-17, 22, 185
   renal failure 19, 197
   strokes 19
prevention
   diabetic retinopathy 201
   hypoglycaemia 73, 96
   long term complications 73-4
   unwanted effects of treatment 73
primary care team
   clinical management of foot ulceration 142-3
   clinical management of hyperglycaemia 108
   education needs 9-15
   education self-help 12
   education syllabus 13-15
   eye care and screening provisions 119-20
   foot care and surveillance provisions 130-1
   materials and resources for 172-4
   role in achieving St Vincent Declaration targets 206
   role in clinical audit and evaluation 165
   role in monitoring and control 106-7
   self-assessment of diabetes knowledge 9-10
priority groups, for chiropody treatment 25
problems, in giving information to patients 146
process measures 166

professional membership, BDA 27, 209
proliferative retinopathy 197, 201
protein restriction in diet, in IDDM 199, 200
proteinuria 198
   testing equipment 40, 198
protocols
   annual reviews 67
   clinical management of foot ulceration 142-3
   diagnosis and management of NIDDM in the normal weight 64
   diagnosis and management of NIDDM in the overweight 63
   dietary treatment 80-1
   distance vision testing 123
   foot examination 134-5
   footwear examination 135
   fundoscopy examination 127-8
   initial assessment of newly diagnosed patients 61-2
   initiating self monitoring programme 113-14
   installing mydriatic drops 127-8
   OGTT 51-2
   routine reviews 65-6
   shoe examination 135
   teaching self administration of insulin 91-8
   visual acuity testing 124-5
psychological factors
   affecting patient education 144-7
   at diagnosis 49, 144
   at initial assessment 61, 62
   hospital referral for psychological problems 65
   insulin therapy 92
public awareness, diabetes 47-8
publishers, addresses 171-2, 174
pyr insulin 89

random blood glucose levels 46, 49, 52
recall and follow up 67-70
    patients with 'at risk' feet 135
receptionists 7, 36
record keeping
    materials and resources 42-3
    organisation 43-4
    practice information 43-4
    recall and follow up 68, 70
    visual acuity testing results 123, 125
    see also practice diabetes register
reinforcement, self monitoring 114
religious factors 99-102
renal failure
    prevalence 19, 197
    progression 198
    see also diabetic nephropathy
renal threshold 49-50
research, BDA funding 27
responsibilities for care provision
    GPs 3
    practice nurses 3
    practice team 3-8
retinopathy see diabetic retinopathy
reviews
    annual 67, 147, 156-7
    DOH requirements 217
    rights and roles of people with
        diabetes 211-12
    routine 65-6, 147
rights and roles, people with diabetes
    210-13
risks
    pregnancy 183, 190
    to feet 131-3
roles in care provision 7
    administrative staff 7-8
    BDA 27-9
    chiropodists 25-6
    diabetologists 23
    dietitians 24-5, 75-6

roles in care provision (continued)
    GPs 3
    nurse specialists 23-4
    people with diabetes 210-13
    practice managers 8
    practice nurses 4-6, 75
    practice team 3-8
    specialist teams 22
routine reviews 65-6
    assessment of self management
        147
Royal College of Nurses 3

St Vincent Declaration
    booklets and leaflets 215, 216
    recommendations for the care of
        children 214-16
    recommendations for clinical audit
        and evaluation 165
    recommendations on driving
        licences, employment and
        insurance 213
    targets xi-xii, 206
salt intake, BDA recommendations 79
screening
    candidates for 48
    equipment 40
    eyes see eye care and screening
    feet see foot care and surveillance
    opportunities 48
secondary diabetes 192-5
self administration of insulin, patient
    education 91-8
self assessment, primary care team's
    knowledge of diabetes 9-10
self management
    assessing candidates 147
    patient education 144-52
self monitoring 113-18
    blood testing 116-18, 183
    diaries 42, 116, 118
    during pregnancy 116, 183

self monitoring (*continued*)
protocol for initiating programme
113-14
reasons for 114-15
urine testing 115-16
serum fructosamine 106
setting up
practice diabetes register 55-6
practice diabetes service 33-44
recall and follow up system 68
shared care 38, 221-2
shoes
examination 135
patient education 139-40, 157
side-effects
guar gum 86
insulin therapy *see* hypoglycaemia
metformin 85
mydriatic drops 127
preventing unwanted effects of
treatments 73
sulphonylureas 84
signs
IDDM 46
NIDDM 46
Sikhs 102, 104
smoking, key information points for
patient education 156
Snellen charts 38, 41, 121
social life
affecting self-management ability
146
key information points for patient
education 156
see also sport and exercise; travel
and holidays
socks *see* footwear
sources, insulin 89
specialist teams
contact names and numbers 42,
56-7
in diabetes centres 26

specialist teams (*continued*)
establishing availability of services
56-8
links with practice diabetes service
34, 36, 56-7
roles in care provision 22
see also individual members by
speciality eg chiropodists
sport and exercise 81, 160-1, 185
starting treatment, insulin therapy
for NIDDM 88
statistics
BDA membership 27
blindness 17, 201
care provision 21-2
costs of diabetes 20
foetal death 183
gestational diabetes 190
impotence 202
long term complications 196
mortality 18-19
practice nurses 4
requirements for insulin therapy for
NIDDM 86
see also clinical audit and evaluation; monitoring and audit;
prevalence
stockings *see* footwear
strokes, prevalence 19
sucrose *see* sugar
sugar, BDA recommendations 80, 181
sulphonylureas 82-4
action 82, 180
combination therapy 86, 186
drug interactions 87
support services, contact names and
numbers 42, 56-7, 60
supra-filtration 198
syllabus, for education of primary
care team 13-15
symptoms
candidates for screening 48

symptoms (*continued*)
  diabetic nephropathy 198
  hyperglycaemia 108
  hypoglycaemia 112
  IDDM 45-6, 182
  NIDDM 45-6, 72, 186
  relieving 72
syringes 93

targets
  glycaemic control 66
  St Vincent Declaration xi-xii, 206
teaching *see* patient education
teenagers *see* young people
teeth *see* dental care
tests
  required at annual reviews 67
  required at initial assessment 62
  required at routine reviews 66
  required for diagnosis 49-52
  see also individually by object of
    test eg visual acuity testing, and
    by type eg urine testing
tetanus immunisation 159
tights *see* footwear
travel and holidays
  insurance 162
  key information points for patient
    education 162-3
  useful addresses 163
treatment of diabetes
  effectiveness 20
  recorded in practice diabetes
    register 56
  rights and roles of people with
    diabetes 210-13
  see also treatment of IDDM;
    treatment of NIDDM
treatment of diabetic retinopathy
  effectiveness 20
  laser therapy 129, 201, 202
treatment of foot ulceration 142-3

treatment of gestational diabetes 190
treatment of hypoglycaemia 112-13
  materials for emergencies 41
  patient education 96
treatment of IDDM 182
treatment of NIDDM
  aims 72-4
  starting treatment 74-5
  see also by type of treatment eg
    insulin therapy
trial period, insulin therapy for
    NIDDM 88, 186
triglyceride levels, testing 62
tumours 192, 193
tuning forks 41, 134

UK Prospective Diabetes Study 27
UKCC 3
ulceration *see* foot ulceration
urine testing
  at annual reviews 67
  at initial assessment 62
  at routine reviews 66
  gestational diabetes 190
  key information points for patient
    education 155
  materials 40, 115-16
  self monitoring 115-16
  use in diabetes diagnosis 49
usage
  guar gum 86
  metformin 85
  sulphonylureas 83-4

vascular disease *see* ischaemia
videos 42, 173, 174
visual acuity testing 120-5, 201, 202
  equipment 41, 121-3
  recording results 123, 125
visual changes, temporary 120-1
vocational driving licences 161-2, 186

WHO
  Health for All programme xii
  OGTT recommendations 51, 186
work *see* employment
World Health Organisation *see* WHO

young people
  care provision 21, 23
  diabetes clinics 21, 61

young people (*continued*)
  key information points for patient
    education 159-60
  prevalence of diabetes 17
  St Vincent Declaration recommen-
    dations 214-16
  services from BDA 28
Youth department, BDA 28